8 Minute Makeovers

CLASSIC

ROMANTIC

EARTHY

GLAMOUR

Be what

you *need* to be—

the woman who

sets the mood

of every occasion.

8 Minute Makeovers

Your Most Beautiful Face For Every Occasion

Clare Miller

ACROPOLIS BOOKS LTD.

WASHINGTON, D.C.

Acknowledgments

I wish to acknowledge my talented co-author, Aleen O'Sullivan, with thanks for all she taught me along the journey to publication; the mentors of my early days, Mulford J. Nobbs and Gerry Tausch; special champions Peggy Miller, Margaret Miller, Gidge Taylor, Bev Walters, Dave Beck, Frank and Paula Little, Laurie Tag, Sandy Trupp, Kathleen Hughes, Robert Hickey, Christopher Jones, Al Hackl, and my staunchest believer and financier, Jerry.

ACROPOLIS BOOKS, LTD.
Colortone Building, 2400 17th St., N.W.,
Washington, D.C. 20009

Printed in the United States of America by
COLORTONE PRESS
Creative Graphics, Inc.
Washington, D.C. 20009

Attention: Schools and Corporations
ACROPOLIS books are available at quantity discounts with bulk purchase for educational, business, or sales promotional use. For information, please write to: SPECIAL SALES DEPARTMENT, ACROPOLIS BOOKS LTD., 2400 17th ST., N.W., WASHINGTON, D.C. 20009

Are there Acropolis Books you want but cannot find in your local stores?
You can get any Acropolis book title in print. Simply send title and retail price, plus 50 cents per copy to cover mailing and handling costs for each book desired. District of Columbia residents add applicable sales tax. Enclose check or money order only, no cash please, to:
ACROPOLIS BOOKS LTD., 2400 17th St., N.W., WASHINGTON, D.C. 20009.

Library of Congress Cataloging in Publication Data

Miller, Clare,
    8 minute makeovers.

    Includes index.
    1. Beauty, Personal. 2. Cosmetics. 3. Face—Care and hygiene. I.Title. Title: Eight minute makeovers.
RA778.M614 1984   646.7'042   84-70406
ISBN 0-87491-736-0

Dedication

To women everywhere,
in search of more
than just beauty.

Contents

You Can Have
4 Different Images
In 8 Minutes!

Image Projection

This is not just a beauty book, it is also a book about image projection. In addition to releasing your loveliest face, you can project a style—or image—to match your mood, your goals, or your setting!

Here are the tricks of makeup and color artistry, hairstyling, and accessorizing, but more importantly, here's how to use those skills quickly, easily, and consistently to create a variety of images—how to put your best, and your prettiest, face forward for every occasion.

Why image projection? Why would you want to go beyond beauty, into style? And what can you achieve with images? You look more interesting, as well as attractive, with style. You add spice to your different moods and activities with family, your special man, friends, and community. You must suit your settings, looking appropriate for office, sports, civic meetings, and evenings out. You gain control of the impression you make, at interviews, social events, on-the-job, in public, at home, wherever. Skillful image projection is a necessary element of living life to the fullest!

Use this book to enhance your *life* as well as your looks. From making that desired "first impression," to mood-setting, your appearance influences the reactions and moods of all those around you. As you know, it has an impact on everything you do and everyone you're with. Your well-chosen image can change your life, and here are 4 fast, sure-fire formulas from which to choose!

You, the modern woman, not only need beauty and style, you also need more than one style from which to choose. Our lifestyles are infinitely more complicated than our mothers' ever were. Each day finds the modern woman giving more than 100% whether she's Supermom, Supersexy, Superachiever. It all adds up to super—demanding!

Because you're so busy, you tend to end up wearing practically the same face with all your clothes and for all your roles—and that one may not have an "image." You'd like your appearance to keep up with you, but you need to be able to change your image quickly, easily, reliably, and excitingly! That's a tall order, but *8 Minute Makeovers* leads the way!

As challenging as your lifestyle is, you're to be praised for learning so well how to wear colors and styles in makeup, hair, and fashion to flatter your natural appearance. You have learned better than any previous generation how to emphasize your good points in order to look your prettiest.

Yet haven't you noticed women no more attractive than you are who somehow manage to look more eye-catchingly interesting and stylish-looking—more "in the know"? If you could just stop and study them, you could figure out the secret combinations that have pulled it all together for them. Their secret is style.

Now you can easily project one or more different images, choosing from the 4 style-producing formulas in this book. Regardless of the occasion or activity, you'll be perfectly confident that your look is appropriate. And, more fun, you'll have some choices of statements—images—to make with your makeup, hairstyle, accessories, and fashions.

Even for an uneventful day, you will find that it takes no more time to use your beauty products in a style than it does to stab on a lipstick and whisk on a blusher in no style. The easiest and fastest image is usually the one that best suits your looks and personality. Since it involves no hard labor or extra time, why not learn to look your very best with your 8 minute—or less!—makeover?

Perhaps you only want to look your prettiest and aren't considering your mood, your goals, or your setting. Choose the image that emphasizes your best features, and presto—you are your prettiest with panache!

Curious about your choices? The 4 image formulas are: Classic, Earthy, Romantic, and Glamour. You can find out which one—or more—of the 4 images best suits your personality, lifestyle, and goals by taking the Image Quiz next.

Don't waste any more time wishing you had your own private makeup artist and hair stylist. These formulas are not hit-or-miss; they work for everybody!

How? When you make up one set of your features to stand out more than the others, you get a specific image. Let's say you have strong eyebrows and wear lots of eye makeup but not much else. Because you're emphasizing your brows and eyes more than the rest of your face, you have created an Earthy Image! Sound easy? It is! This balance of power, decided by where you put your makeup emphasis, creates your style.

Do you wonder where these formulas come from? We have our "foremothers" to thank. They developed the 4 distinct styles, now tailored to your modern use, that can be yours using the formulas in this book. Let's take a ride through Celebrity Land, to get a feeling for the Classic, Earthy, Romantic, and Glamour Images:

Queens Cleopatra and Nefertiti of Egypt projected the Glamour Image (emphasis on eyes and lips, and the use of strong colors).

The ladies of Regency England (the 1800's), who were neither outspoken nor openly aggressive, captured the essence of romance. Theirs was the Romantic Image (a soft, rosy, "no makeup" look).

Clara Bow, of the famous lips, and Ruby Keeler are symbolic of the early 1900's, when women reasserted their freedom to wear obvious makeup. They epitomized a romantic kind of Glamour, as women eased their way back into a somewhat bolder beauty using a bit more cosmetic help.

By the 1930's women had the vote, and the nerve to smolder in very high Glamour indeed. Marlene Dietrich, Greta Garbo, and Joan Crawford smouldered with the best of them!

Later, Greer Garson, Gene Tierney, Olivia de Havilland, Maggie Smith, and Katharine Hepburn revived the classical theme of ancient Greece and Rome. The postwar 1940's and 1950's brought a new return to elegance: the

Classic Image (eyebrow, cheekbone, lip emphasis), which cleverly copied the high standards of ancient times.

Initially, Natalie Wood, Jackie O., Lena Horne, Kim Novak, Elke Sommer, and Jane Fonda reflected the relaxed standards of the 1960's, which gave birth to a sophisticated Earthy Image never seen before. With our new urban brand of sophistication, we sported sharply-defined eyeliner, false eyelashes, and teased, bouffant hair. Lips were whited-out to de-emphasize them. Earthy Image (eyebrow, eye, and hair emphasis) isn't necessarily "natural" looking!

Sophia Loren, Julie Christie, and Raquel Welch followed with a more subtle version of this glamorous Earthy image. As we progressed into the 60's, gentle "flower children" and outspoken feminists alike shared the spotlight. Glamorous Earthy gave way to the demand for au naturel, and developed into a natural Earthy Image closer to the Original Image: a Garden of Eden naturalness, with strong eyebrows and eyes, typified by Ali McGraw and Goldie Hawn.

In an historic first, the 1970's brought the dual reign of two images: Earthy and Glamour. Earthy examples include Farrah Fawcett, Cheryl Tiegs, and Jacqueline Bisset. Among the glamour stars include: Ann-Margret and Cher.

In the enlightened 1980's, we see women using all the images, from Glamour and Romantic to Earthy and Classic. Today's beauty celebrities are more interesting and memorable because they're not committed to a single image. The striking Meryl Streep, Nastassia Kinski, Shari Belafonte, Jaclyn Smith, Barbra Streisand, Shelley Duvall, Glenda Jackson and Lynda Carter are among the many who could be put into time-capsules and enjoyed in any millennium.

Your Self-Discovery

Now let's talk about you. First take the Image Quiz to discover which images suit your personality, lifestyle, and goals. From your quiz answers, pick the one that sounds like the right one for your plans today, and turn to the chapter in the book devoted to that image. You will read briefly about how this look benefits you, and where/when you should wear it. Then step up to the mirror and try it on!

In the back of the book are quick-reference Fast Face tear-out sheets. Remove the Fast Face tear-sheet for the image you have chosen and put it up near your mirror. This is your easy, step-by-step formula for your 8-minute makeover (you may need a little longer the first time).

Before you begin your makeover, be sure you've "prepared the canvas" with good skin care. (There is a special skin-care section included in the book). Now apply your tailored-to-the-image makeup, as illustrated on the Fast Face pin-up. You probably have on hand a little of everything you need. (Anything you're missing can be easily purchased).

You've finished your makeover? Congratulations! You are no longer a face without an image! You may now go back to your image chapter. After the Fast Face section there, you'll see The Total Look chart. Check that chart for any guidance you'd like on colors, hairstyle, accessories, and the general overview of your image. Skim through the Check-Out, which follows, to be sure you've pulled it all together.

If you'd like more detail on colors, hair, and accessories for that image, just keep turning the pages of that chapter! You'll find information for the serious color student, keyed to the popular terminology of *Color Me Beautiful* and *Alive with Color* (Acropolis Books), and "Color 1." Lastly, the Model Face section of the chapter gives you more detail for makeup for occasions when you have the time and inclination to go "all out" on your face.

If you have any special considerations—good skin care; a facial feature you wish to improve with makeup contouring; an evening-light makeup adjustment; altered hair color; eyeglasses; photogenic makeup—you may want to refer to those special sections in the book. The special sections, however, are not a must in creating an image. Each image formula is already complete in its own chapter.

Your Image Quiz

Settle back and enjoy this quiz. There are no right or wrong answers! They will all help you pick out your current top favorites from among the 4 images, and the quiz works best if you don't spend any time on your answers.

Just "x" the one answer (or two, if it's a toss-up) that appeals to you most after your first *QUICK* scan.

1. You're choosing a color for a special dressing gown. It would be:
   a ☐ a flattering medium or dark neutral
   b ☐ a bright red
   c ☐ a soft green
   d ☐ a becoming light pink

2. Your rich uncle has found four boats he thinks you will like. He would like to give you one to have when you need to get away. You would choose:
   a ☐ a fishing boat
   b ☐ a small sailboat
   c ☐ a houseboat
   d ☐ a speed boat

3. You're offered a chance to practice dancing with an expert. You choose:
   a ☐ ballet
   b ☐ square dancing
   c ☐ jazz dancing
   d ☐ ballroom dancing

4. Your hairdresser has promised you he can create any hairstyle you'd like to coordinate with your wedding gown. On your head you choose to wear:
   a ☐ flowers entwined in your hair
   b ☐ a pearl-embroidered Juliet cap and cathedral veil
   c ☐ a high-style, wide-brimmed hat
   d ☐ veiling held in place by an antique comb

5. A wealthy friend has come into your life and wants to impress you. Knowing your taste in art, your friend buys you a priceless:
   a ☐ French Impressionist painting
   b ☐ ancient Greek marble sculpture
   c ☐ Picasso painting
   d ☐ ancient work of Indian art

6. You haven't seen your special man in several months. He reappears, and you make plans to meet for dinner later in the week. Would you prefer:
   a ☐ an intimate dinner at home by candlelight
   b ☐ a sunset dinner picnic for two at the lake
   c ☐ supper at your private club, which has a stunning disco underneath
   d ☐ dinner at that quiet restaurant where only he has ever taken you

7. You are building your dream home, in which you'll reside for most of the year. Your architect brings you four plans, knowing you'll flip over one in particular. He's right, and you make your decision immediately. He felt sure your favorite was going to be:
   a ☐ an ivy-covered Tudor cottage
   b ☐ a contemporary home by Frank Lloyd Wright
   c ☐ a California ranch-style home
   d ☐ an elegant colonial townhome

8. You would describe one of your favorite fragrances as:
   a ☐ crisp, clean, and spicy or quietly cosmopolitan
   b ☐ sweetly lingering, softly feminine; maybe floral
   c ☐ casual, woodsy, mellow; or musky, deep, primeval
   d ☐ sparkling, elegant, lightly mysterious

9. You are trained for all of the following careers. Your first choice is:
   a ☐ show-animal trainer
   b ☐ United Nations interpreter
   c ☐ museum curator
   d ☐ corporate attorney

10. If you could only belong to one, you would choose:
    a ☐ swim and aerobics spa
    b ☐ tennis and hunt club
    c ☐ debate and drama club
    d ☐ iceskaters club

11. You have a great figure and can wear anything. You know your man's favorite color is red, so on a formal occasion you wear a red:
    a ☐ slinky, sequin gown cut low in front and back
    b ☐ floor-length chiffon trimmed with ruffles at the v-neck and wrists
    c ☐ shimmery form-molded sheath with manderin collar and slits up both sides
    d ☐ velvet blazer and skirt, with contrasting silk blouse tied at the neck with a bow

12. You have never taken any of the free classes available at your community college. They are offering a one-time-only chance for you to take them with world-renowned masters. You sign up for:
    a ☐ jewelry design and creation; baking
    b ☐ furniture repair; healthy gourmet cookery
    c ☐ silk-screening; entertainment foods
    d ☐ furniture refinishing; natural foods cookery

13. You're single and would like to join another of those classes as a lark to see if you can meet a man there who's your type. So you also sign up for:
    a ☐ small-craft pilot training
    b ☐ public speaking and media communications
    c ☐ financial planning and budget management
    d ☐ travel, photography and journalism

14. It's extremely hot, and you want to put your hair up for a lunch with friends. It's medium length and could be worn:
    a ☐ in a Gibson-girl topknot with escaped wisp curls
    b ☐ off the face in front with a tidy tortoise hairband
    c ☐ sleekly pulled back into a shiny severe chignon
    d ☐ all up in a "tail" at the back with a large clip

15. You are going to a lavish costume party and your escort has offered you carte blanche at a costume-rental emporium. You choose to go as:
    a ☐ a countess
    b ☐ a shepherdess
    c ☐ a Hawaiian girl
    d ☐ a flamenco dancer

16. Of the four, this trip would be your all-time favorite:
    a ☐ A sunny Caribbean cruise
    b ☐ Paris in the spring
    c ☐ The British Isles in tweed
    d ☐ A bite out of the Big Apple: New York City

17. Which would you like to have the most of during your lifetime?
    a ☐ fame
    b ☐ money
    c ☐ knowledge
    d ☐ love

18. The images you most need to project to others are:
    a ☐ successful, understated, refined, authority
    b ☐ sparkling, avant garde, exciting, mysterious
    c ☐ soft, spontaneous, feminine, youthful, innocent
    d ☐ natural, physical, informal, carefree, sensual

19. Your current hair color is:
   a ☐ ash, platinum, silver, or white blond
   b ☐ strawberry blonde or strawberry red
   c ☐ golden, honey, or flaxen blonde or warm grey
   d ☐ silver, salt-and-pepper, charcoal grey, or white
   e ☐ auburn or carrot red
   f ☐ chestnut or coppery red-brown
   g ☐ light taupe or "mouse," medium brown
   h ☐ dishwater blonde, or brown with strawberry hints
   i ☐ dark brown
   j ☐ brown-black
   k ☐ blue-black
   l ☐ champagne frosted or ash frosted
   m ☐ sunny, or sun-streaked hair

20. Your naturally best and strongest features are:
   a ☐ eyebrows and eyes
   b ☐ complexion and curvy face
   c ☐ eyes and lips
   d ☐ eyebrows, cheekbones, lips

21. You usually spend this much time on your face and hair:
   a ☐ almost none
   b ☐ a little
   c ☐ a medium amount
   d ☐ a lot

22. Your current status is:
   a ☐ Age 11
   b ☐ Age 11-17
   c ☐ Age 17-22, student
   d ☐ Age 17-22, in professional life
   e ☐ Age 22-35, at home
   f ☐ Age 22-35, in professional life
   g ☐ Age 35-45
   h ☐ Age 45-55, with well cared-for skin
   i ☐ Age 45-55, with well cared-for skin, in professional life
   j ☐ Age 45-55, with weathered skin
   l ☐ Age 55-65, with well cared-for skin
   m ☐ Age 55-65, with weathered skin
   n ☐ Over 65

Now add up your answers and discover the image you should be wearing to match your moods!

Answers to Your Image Quiz

Circle the image that matches your answer to each of the questions.

1. a. Classic
   b. Glamour
   c. Earthy
   d. Romantic

2. a. Earthy
   b. Classic
   c. Romantic
   d. Glamour

3. a. Romantic
   b. Earthy
   c. Glamour
   d. Classic

4. a. Earthy
   b. Classic
   c. Glamour
   d. Romantic

5. a. Romantic
   b. Classic
   c. Glamour
   d. Earthy

6. a. Classic
   b. Earthy
   c. Glamour
   d. Romantic

7. a. Romantic
   b. Glamour
   c. Earthy
   d. Classic

8. a. Classic
   b. Romantic
   c. Earthy
   d. Glamour

9. a. Earthy
   b. Glamour
   c. Romantic
   d. Classic

10. a. Earthy
    b. Classic
    c. Glamour
    d. Romantic

11. a. Glamour
    b. Romantic
    c. Earthy
    d. Classic

12. a. Romantic
    b. Classic
    c. Glamour
    d. Earthy

13. a. Earthy
    b. Glamour
    c. Classic
    d. Romantic

14. a. Romantic
    b. Classic
    c. Glamour
    d. Earthy

15. a. Classic
    b. Romantic
    c. Earthy
    d. Glamour

16. a. Earthy
    b. Romantic
    c. Classic
    d. Glamour

17. a. Glamour
    b. Classic
    c. Earthy
    d. Romantic

18. a. Classic
    b. Glamour
    c. Romantic
    d. Earthy

Question 19.
Your hair color looks best in these images:
(next best in parentheses, in preference order)
a. Classic (and Glamour)
b. Romantic (and Earthy)
c. Romantic (and Classic, Earthy, Glamour)
d. Glamour or Classic
e. Romantic (and Earthy, Classic, Glamour)
f. Earthy (Romantic, Classic, Glamour)
g. Classic (and Earthy, Romantic)
h. Classic (and Romantic, Earthy)
i. Classic (and Glamour, Romantic)
j. Classic or Glamour (and Romantic)
k. Glamour (and Classic, Romantic, Earthy)
l. Classic (and Glamour)
m. Earthy (and Classic, Romantic, Glamour)

Question 20
    a. Earthy
    b. Romantic
    c. Glamour
    d. Classic

Question 21
    a. Earthy
    b. Romantic
    c. Classic
    d. Glamour

Question 22
Certain images suit certain ages particularly well:

a. 11 . . . . Romantic
b. 11-17 . . . . Romantic, Earthy
c. 17-22 Student . . . . . . Classic, Romantic, Earthy, Glamour
d. 17-22 Professional . . Classic during work hours + Romantic, Earthy, Glamour off-hours
e. 22-35 . . . . Classic, Romantic, Earthy, Glamour
f. 22-35 Professional . . Classic during work hours + Romantic, Earthy, Glamour off-hours
g. 35-45 . . . . Classic, Romantic, Glamour
h. 45-55 Good Skin . . . Classic, Romantic, Glamour
i. 45-55 Good Skin, Professional
    Classic during work hours + Romantic, Glamour off-hours
j. 45-55 Weathered . . . Classic
k. 55-65 Good Skin . . . Classic, Romantic, Glamour
l. 55-65 Weathered . . . Classic
m. Over 65 . . . . Romantic, Glamour

Now add up your circled images:

Earthy . . . . = ☐

Romantic . . . . = ☐

Glamour . . . . = ☐

Classic . . . . = ☐

The Images I Should Start to Wear, Because They Are Most Suited to My Personality, Lifestyle, & Goals:

I scored high on _____ Image.

I also like to wear (2nd) _____ Image.

(3rd) _____ Image.

(4th) _____ Image.

I didn't score this time in _____ Image.

(Important note: If your answer to Question 20 is one of these images, that image best suits the appearance you were born with. You will want to wear it on days when you don't have a particular mood or goal—and just want to look your prettiest with style.)

Now you want to try out your first image, right? Take a look at the color plates to get a feeling for what the images look like, and then head straight for the chapter of your choice to find out how easy they are to achieve! Good luck!

And don't forget to come back to this Image Quiz once in a while and take it again. As you mature and change, your needs—and your taste in styles—will change too.

Chapter 1

The
Classic
Face

Setting The Mood

Can you remember—or reconstruct by catching several TV late shows—the graceful appeal of the leading actresses of the 1940's, particularly the American breed? If so, you will instantly grasp the character of the statement (or, in this case, understatement) you will make wearing your Classic Face.

The elements comprising this classically beautiful image—the Classic Face—are not outdated. More than any other beauty style, this one exemplifies the American Dream: the image of winning, riches, and success without compromise. The aura is one of elegance and refinement; wealth, power and assurance; quality and integrity; understatement and timelessness.

How Did The Classic Image Become So Popular?

During the 1940's, World War II made rationing a part of everyone's life. Paring down to essentials was the model of the day. Strength was demanded of everyone; men were soldiering, and women left their homes to join every area of the labor force—a first in our western culture.

Women, worldwide, now held a permanently significant role in two camps: the family unit, and the traditionally male-dominated civic and career world.

In such a climate of change, the internationally accepted style of beauty changed, too. It mellowed, from overtly glamorous into a subtle image that radiated competence yet maintained grace, and self-assurance. The perception of beauty grew from the single "hothouse" beauty image, attainable only by the elite, to an aura of self-confidence accessible to the middle classes.

Famous Classic Faces

An image to match the mood of that era evolved most vividly in Hollywood, where the makeup artists of the 40's and 50's began to emphasize the sculptured, symmetrical features of the American beauties of the day. Classic constellations you will recognize include Gene Tierney, Irene Dunne, Greer Garson, Maggie Smith, and Katharine Hepburn.

Nearly every great actress of modern times has also worn this image for some role, simply because the strength of that classical style has left such a powerful impact on our concept of beauty. Today the basic components of this image are still regarded by American eyes, and those of many other nations, as the key elements of refined beauty.

Because Olivia de Havilland, Diahann Carroll, the late Princess Grace of Monaco, and First Lady Nancy Reagan felt that this face projected their personality so well, they have worn it exclusively, and a classic style has become synonymous with their public image.

Almost every woman has wanted to wear, at some time, this ultimate "American Beauty Face" for the look that is still regarded as the most "civilized".

Why and When Do You Wear the Classic Image?

Aren't there times when you're not sure where you'll be going, what you'll be doing, or with whom you'll be doing it? At times like these, you really appreciate having the Classic Image at your command. It's like a security blanket in which you can wrap yourself, knowing that you are appropriately dressed no matter where you go.

In fact, Classic Image exudes such an aura of timeless beauty and style that if you want to stick with a single image and never vary it, Classic is the one to choose. Classic never appears dated or outdated, since it doesn't utilize current fads and trends.

When you need to assure the world of your wisdom or wealth, bring on Classic Face—the one that never lets you down.

When you need to get people behind you to get something done—whether for yourself or for a cause—it's important to create an image of success and authority. No one feels motivated about backing something new by someone who doesn't appear to be in control. And Classic Image shows self-control, which is a good start!

That same "discipline" about your appearance is what makes Classic Image the perfect one for your professional needs. You're reflected as a disciplined winner at your workplace or whatever else you're taking on. It gives you the look of the type who, when under pressure or fire, is coolly competent. Because none of the other images has this unique quality, you owe it to yourself and the people you're working with to wear Classic consistently during your professional hours.

Women in business have long understood that the Classic image is the success-producing style. It's much easier to sell that million-dollar house if you look like you're at ease around millions and might, in fact, live in such a house yourself! The "Career Woman" cameo at the end of this Classic Image chapter will ice the Classic cake of your working hours.

Where Do You Wear the Classic Image

Now that you know why and when to choose your Classic look, here are some times and places—both rare and not-so-rare—for wearing it.

As a participant or a spectator, Classic is a must when you are involved in any of such affluent leisure sports as swimming, tennis, golf, skiing (on water or snow), biking, horseback riding, squash, sailing, polo, rugby, lacrosse, or most strenuous of all—tailgate parties and sport-booster clubs! Sorry if your pet favorite has been left off the list; there are so many. Just add it yourself, and don your Classic.

Are you about to go on an interview, and trying hard not to bite the very fingernails you'd like to have look their best when you make that good first impression? Classic Image takes the worry out of your appearance, whether it's a corporate job interview, or any other interview where you need a success image. It may not guarantee you the job, but with Classic you'll know your appearance didn't hold you back. Good luck!

Let your capability gain credibility in your own business office, in the "other guy's" office, and at special meetings called in restaurants and other public places. Don't let down your Classic guard with the change of scene.

You'll thrill to business travel with Classic Image. It's so easy to pack, and light, because everything coordinates, and fast because you don't have to stand around trying to decide what looks you need. With Classic, it's clear-cut. And the best part is you know you'll look right when you get there. Seminars, conventions, company get-togethers—whip out your Classic look wherever you need to put your best foot forward.

You won't want to be considered a slouch when you represent the family on "state occasions."Often the family and friends present at these gatherings haven't seen you in a while, and we're all human enough to want to look as though we've made progress since the last meeting. It's especially important when these functions are solemn and meaningful to don your most refined Classic look. Remember Classic for church-going, family (and school) reunions, christenings, graduations, marriages, and funerals.

Are you having your picture taken? For passports, yearbooks, publicity, portraits, or posterity: Classic gives predictable results and won't embarrass you later! (Don't forget to add a bit of photogenic wizardry from the camera tips section in this book.)

Civic and social organization meetings are not the right settings for your warm-up suit. You'll be sure to see a hundred people you didn't expect to be there, including the boss and his wife, or that potential client you are trying to land. One word of warning—don't wear your professional-best Classic unless you want to get elected to leadership at PTA meetings, town hall meetings, church socials, or neighborhood planning meetings.

Are your palms sweating as you prepare for a visit to court, or are you hoping to convince a judge to see that parking ticket your way? Do you want to seem wise in jury duty, be a great help to your favorite political crusades' fundraisers and campaigns, and look correct for other governmental gatherings? Vote for Classic.

When you're heading for libraries, museums, art galleries, parades, tourist sight-seeing, historical vacation sites, or country homes, Classic's aura is likely to be the mood you want to convey. Any of these outings tend to be more comfortable when you wear Classic, and comfort can become more and more important as the day wears on!

Even if you're one who traditionally chooses Glamour for art galleries, evening concerts and ballets—or Earthy for parades and athletic competitions—a switch to Classic once in a while keeps you from becoming bored with your preferred image, and predictable. (By the way, you can shimmer in Classic with a minor adjustment for after-5:00 light.) So for a posh concert, ballet, opera, play, restaurant, or club, the Classic you is a charming addition to any party.

An extra scoop of pleasure is added to life when you really get going with the theme of your setting. Try your most easy-going Classic Image for your "gentry sporting life": country clubs, resorts, getaways, log cabins and lodges out in the countryside, British-flavor nightclubs, pubs and of course St. Patrick's Day celebrations.

Whenever you're in uniform, Classic is automatic—with no deviation. The very purpose of a uniform is one of the goals of Classic Image: to inspire trust in your discipline, strength, control, and winning abilities.

Speaking of uniforms, Classic Image is perfect to get you into, and help you fit in, boarding schools, prep schools, and military schools. The unofficial uniform of sororities and fraternities is definitely Classic. And speaking of schools, colleges and universities never object when you apply for admission in Classic Image, nor does it hurt your grades to show up for class wearing Classic.

Are you single, dating, and hoping to marry "old money" or name? Having Classic Image in your "old kit bag" can give you an edge. Some men lean toward Glamour and Earthy Images; but "old money" tends to find understatement more alluring. Yes, Virginia, there really are men who prefer women in kilts and kneesocks! You're the kind they want to take home to mother.

Are you planning to vacation in Boston, on Nantucket or Cape Cod, in Virginia and Washington, D.C.—or in other strongholds East Coast and deep South? Or perhaps in the British Isles? It might be fun to be taken (mistaken?) for a Classic, even though you've just donned the look for the trip.

Do you need to win something badly? Your appearance may give you a leg up. It can sway the judges and add credibility and importance to your entry. It can also intimidate the competition. (I asked if you wanted to win badly, remember?) Best of all, it psychs you up to that attitude of feeling in control, in the winner mode, and razor's edge ready.

Athletic competitions, business quotas and challenges, singles mixers, skill competitions, political races, dog shows, dance competitions, beauty pageants (the interview), talent shows, Guinness record-setting…in the great American way, the list is endless and our winners legion. And you supporters of those competitors contribute, too, so sport that Classic Image yourself!

Last but not least are the parties where you'll want to display Classic Image, especially parties celebrating promotions, honors, debutantes, achievements, charitable fundraising, and winnings—to name but a few—of the wonderful reasons for having a party.

What Are the Characteristics of the Classic Face?

What secret beauty formula enabled the women of the 40's to achieve such an aura of grace and elegance that their image became a beauty cornerstone?

They simply echoed a style historically valued: the beauty formula depicted by the old masters of the Renaissance, especially Michelangelo, daVinci, and Corot. These artists created a vision of classic elegance that has retained its validity since the 14th century:

- the classic triangle of symmetrical and well-defined features—eyebrow, cheekbone, and lip;
- pale, unflawed skin;
- opaque, and only medium-intensity colors; and
- oval and angular face shapes.

(Don't lose heart! If you don't have these features, you can create the impression that you do, with cosmetics.)

The old masters combined these elements to create a timeless—and thus modern—elegance that fashion leaders of the 40's worked hard to duplicate. You, however, with today's range of cosmetic tools and know-how at your fingertips, can reproduce this image with far greater ease.

Introducing You to the Classic Image Formula

Do I Have Time for It?

Do you simply put on some lipstick and go, because you're afraid that creating a style will take too much time—time you need for other things? As you can see from the list of activities appropriate for your Classic look, this image is for busy people and can be created quickly!

Wearing nothing but lipstick is like framing half of a picture; the look is terribly unbalanced and unfinished—almost worse than no makeup at all! Especially when you can smooth on a few cosmetics in the Classic formula—in 8 minutes or less—and dash off to enjoy yourself (and be enjoyed) all the more for being attractively styled for the occasion.

Remember—you don't need a lot of time or complicated cosmetic products. You just need a few basic items and a few minutes. What makes the difference—between having no style and having a pretty and Classic style—is that this time you've applied those common makeup items to the right places on your face!

Another plus is that the cosmetics you use in Classic Face are not faddish. There's no need to constantly shop for trendy replacements or wonder which cosmetics to use from your bewildering home collection.

Although you can use many up-to-the-minute colors and products, you will find that, more than the other 4 images, Classic Face resists a trendy appearance. The steps of Classic Face are best completed with basic, middle-range beauty tools, tools that have endured from the earliest days of widespread cosmetics usage. You probably have these on hand already, or can easily find them at a nearby cosmetics counter.

Does Classic Image Work For Me?

Whether or not you have naturally "classic" looks, you can easily achieve this Face. Everybody has eyebrows, cheeks, and lips to emphasize; a little makeup and brow-grooming in the Classic Formula do the rest. If you have irregular features, you may use more makeup—in the Classic Formula—to contour some Classic features for yourself. Classic Face doesn't require a "no-makeup" look.

Face Shapes: Aren't you happy that Classic Face does not need birthright features of thick dark eyebrows, long dark eyelashes, full lips, dainty nose, big eyes, or a complexion so well cared for that it hardly requires correction? However, Classic is easier if you have an oval or one of the angular face shapes: square, rectangle (oblong), triangle (pear), or inverted triangle (heart).

Coloring: We are also lucky that Classic adapts easily to the four color keys (also described here by their popular names): warm, yellow-based (*"Spring/Light-Bright/Sunlight,* and *Fall/Muted/Sunset"*), and cool, blue-based (*"Summer/Gentle/Sunlight,* and *Winter/Contrast/Sunrise"*). Select medium-intensity colors from within your own color key.

If you have light, mild looks (*"Spring, Summer* or *delicate Autumn"*), you are lovelier in Classic than in any of the other images except Romantic. If your coloring is medium-to-strong, cool (*"Winter"*), yet non-dramatic, you have an easy time with Classic, especially the Classic Career Woman. If you have warm, cloudy coloring (*"Autumn/Muted/Sunset"*), you can easily find your medium-range cosmetic colors.

Skin Type: The entire range of natural skin tones and types can project this ageless aura. To appear your palest and most unflawed, use foundation one shade lighter than your current complexion, and blemish concealer if necessary. Powder gives the desirable matte (non-shiny) finish.

The look of suntan says carefree Earthy Image, not Classic. If you like to project a Classic style most of the time, avoid tanning. If you're a dyed-in-the-wool sunworshipper, moisturizers and pale foundations can help when you want the Classic look.

Ages: Although women of every age can successfully wear this face, the youngest set is not usually interested in acquiring what this face achieves; it's thus often not chosen until one reaches the mid-twenties or early thirties.

Eyebrows, Cheekbones, Lips: The triangle of these three features dominates the Classic Face.

And in Classic Face, these three dominant features are created equal! No one of the three features overpowers the other two: the eyebrows are just as strong and attention grabbing as the cheekbones, and the cheekbones are as eye-catching as the lips.

To summarize the basics for creating your Classic Face:
- complexion—your palest, most flawless-looking, matte;
- eyebrows—tidy, arched, emphasized;
- cheekbones—rouged, angular, emphasized;
- lips—sharply-defined, colorful, emphasized; and
- colors—opaque, and medium-intensity.

Classic Fast Face

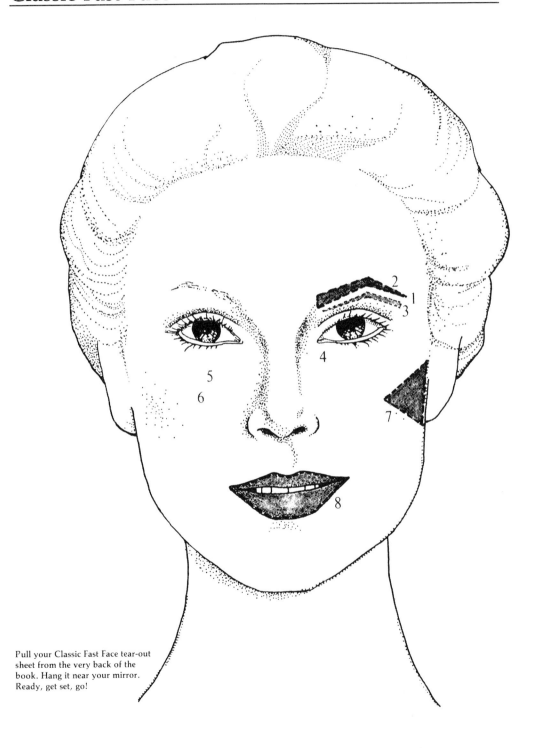

Pull your Classic Fast Face tear-out sheet from the very back of the book. Hang it near your mirror. Ready, get set, go!

Ready to Try Classic Face?

Whether you use the Fast Face or the Model Face makeover, the more closely you follow this classic-appeal blueprint, the more people will believe that you are polished, assured, refined, and successful—from their very first glance.

—Fast Face—Classic Formula

Complexion, Eyebrow, Cheekbone, Lip

Eyebrow

1 Shape, with cake eyebrow powder, into Classic Arch
2 Brush brow, and run the eyebrow brush along top of brow to return any wild hairs back to brow
3 Highlight underneath eyebrow, its full length

Complexion

4 Perfect it: cover circles, blemishes, flaws (and lighten top eyelid centers) with light concealer stick
5 Apply light foundation with makeup sponge

Cheekbones

6 Dust face with a pad of translucent powder (loose, or pressed compact)
7 Brush powder blusher into cheek hollows; blend with sponge

Lips

8 Add opaque, medium lip color—inside, or up to, lip line

Optional Touches

- A light coat of mascara
- Medium eye color in crease of the eye (just above lid)
- Lipliner pencil inside lip line (before lip color)
- Extra whisk (and later touch-ups) with face powder pad

The Total Look

Pulling It All Together for Classic Image

1. Perfect-as-possible skin characterizes the Classic Face: its color is as light as you can manage and usually in the alabaster, lighter-than-skin-tones beige or ivory family. All flaws visually corrected as much as possible. Complexion has fine-pored, matte finish.

2. The three most dominant features in the face are: eyebrows, cheekbones, and lips, specializing in the precise Classic Arched Eyebrow.

3. Classic is characterized by medium, opaque colors.

4. The eyelids tend to be light in color for day-wear, lashes clean and tidy.

5. All features are well-sculpted and as angular as possible.

Eyebrows: arching, angular
1. Classic arch, with highlighter below
2. Self-contained; no stray hairs
3. Evenly filled; not dramatically thick, thin, or round

Cheekbones: sculpted, not rounded
1. Cheekbone flush, with highlighter above
2. The hollow under cheekbone contoured, from temple toward lip
3. Blusher no closer to nose than the pupil of the eye

Lips
1. Symmetrical, sharply defined
2. Medium lip color, no high gloss
3. Lipliner

Hair
1. Upswept or medium-length; shoulder-skimming or above
2. Center, focal point; or side part
3. Long bangs: straight, or in face-framing waves
4. Clean, sleek, smooth-styled, shiny, healthy, neat, symmetrical

Complexion
1. Pale
2. Flawless-looking
3. Matte

Eye Makeup
1. Minimal

Ornaments
1. Tailored
2. Non-dangly, not oversize
3. Not too dramatic

Garments
1. Conservative
2. Tailored
3. Refined
4. Neat, "non-fussy," understated

Buzz Words
1. Brows/Cheeks/Lips
2. Refined, understated
3. Traditional, regular
4. Even, symmetrical
5. Conservative, clean
6. Medium colors, styles
7. Nails not long, showy
8. Fragrance: Crisp, light floral/spice

Check It Out, and Go!

Is my foundation too dark? Or uneven anywhere? Are there any shiny patches, or uncovered blemishes?

Are the eyebrows classically arched and matched? No wild hairs, or gaps in the brow that need filling in? And are my brows just as strong as my cheeks and lips?

Do my cheekbones need a hint more hollowing with blusher? Or just a little more blending with sponge? And are the cheeks just as strong as brows and lips?

How about my lips? Is each side its mirror image? Not too dark or light not to full or glossy? And just as strong as brows and cheeks?

Do my eyes stand out too much?

If you pass your check-out, your statement is one of refined assurance. Isn't it great to feel you could stroll elegantly through a presentation in the boardroom!

This is your winning face, so grab that aura and expect success!

The Classic Color Palette

To create a classic look, your best color choices are opaque rather than sheer and shimmery. They are of medium intensity rather than strongly dark or light.

Your "coolest" colors are best, and your brightest colors or palest pastels are least desirable for Classic. Neutrals, singly or combined, are a sure Classic.

All types of natural coloring can easily create a classic mood.

Think medium, opaque, true, and traditional.

Some Suggested Colors

True navy
True green
Snow white
Steel or charcoal grey
True blue
Emerald green
Primary yellow
True red
Ruby red
Flannel grey
Blue-red
Brown-black

Light, clear navy
Medium spring green
French vanilla
Yellow grey
Light aquamarine
Medium clear turquoise
Banana
Warm shell pink
Any clear coral
Clear camel
Clear tan
Cheese whip

Burgundy
Cordovan
Wine
Maroon
Amethyst
Porcelain rose
Light lemon yellow
Light slate
Wedgwood blue
Heather blue
Heather purple
Lavender grey

Scarlet rust
Dusky geranium
Taupe camel
Dark khaki
Greige (grey-beige)
Light old gold
Cadet blue
Hunter green
Oatmeal
Natural
Very dark brown

Classic Sample Makeup Color Schemes

True Red Scheme

Concealer: "Vert"—cool, blue-green (white) base.

Foundation: Cool—"rachelle"; "rose"; ebony beige tone lighter than skin tone

Face Powder: Lightest, translucent (no frost)

Highlighter: White, light

Creme Rouge: Blue-red, or clear, cool, medium pink

Powder Blush: (contour) True red, or deep, clear medium rose

Lip Pencil: Clear apple, true red, or fuchsia

Lipstick: True reds, bright plum, hot reds, or bright burgundy

Mascara: Bright black

Eye Shadow: True (non-pastel!) blues, true greens, silver grey, or charcoal

Hot Coral Scheme

Concealer: Light, warm, yellow-based

Foundation: Light, warm, yellow-based, ivory lighter than skin tone

Face Powder: Lightest, translucent (no frost)

Highlighter: Light cream or ivory

Creme Rouge: Flame, coral, clear, hot, light pink, or clear bright red

Powder Blush: (contour) Clear, warm, medium coral, or clear, warm, medium pink

Lip Pencil: Clear, warm, medium coral

Lipstick: Clear, warm, medium coral pink or poppy, or flame

Mascara: Soft, bright black

Eye Shadow: Clear, warm, medium coral powder blush, clear, warm spring green, or clear, warm turquoise, honey or amber

For the information of the serious color student:

Clear, Cold, Blue-based (Winter/Contrast/Sunrise)

Clear, Warm, Yellow-based (Spring/Light-Bright/Sunlight)

Sample Makeup Color Schemes

Burgundy Scheme

Concealer: Soft, "off-white"

Foundation: Cool—"rachelle"; "rose"; "ivory bisque;" or beige lighter than skin tone

Face Powder: Lightest, translucent (no frost)

Highlighter: Soft, "off-white"

Creme Rouge: Muted rose, muted burgundy, carnation

Powder Blush (contour): Dusty, cool rose, blue-red

Lip Pencil: Dusty, cool—raspberry/berry/red

Lipstick: Smoky, cool—plum/berry/blue-red

Mascara: Hazy blue-black

Eye Shadow: Soft, medium blue pink-n-rosy mocha, blue-greys, French blue

Bright Rust Scheme

Concealer: Warm, lighter than skin; "oyster" family; warm beige

Foundation: Warm, lighter than skin; "oyster;" warm beige, warm, muted medium ivory

Face Powder: Lightest, translucent (no frost)

Highlighter: Oyster, warm greyed beige

Creme Rouge: Tomato, brick, bright rust, red-orange, orange-red

Powder Blush (contour): cinnamon, warm, medium mahogany, rust

Lip Pencil: Apricot, cinnamon, dusky geranium

Lipstick: Salmon rose, ginger, tomato red, dark red-orange

Mascara: Hazy brown-black, earthy dark brown

Eye Shadow: Loden green, khaki, hunter green, sand, coffee, light, warm mahogany, cadet blue, taupe, muted camel

For the information of the serious color student:

Cloudy, Cool, Blue-based (Summer/Gentle/Sunlight)

Cloudy, Warm, Yellow-based (Autumn/Muted/Sunset)

Classic Hair

Hair designs that present the most classic appeal reflect refined simplicity. Look back to the styles worn by women of the 1940's; you'll see some common trends.

There are no styles more elegant in feeling than those that can be described as "upswept," a style particularly suited to long or medium-length hair. The chignon, the French twist, and the Psyche knot are all synonymous with classic elegance.

Many short hairstyles for women create a controlled, and sometimes even upswept, impression.

Curls from a permanent, straight hair, or thick, slightly wavy hair can all look very neatly sculpted when short.

Whether it's long or short, hair that's unruly, wild, dangling, tousled, pixie, Rive Gauche, generously swirling, or otherwise exaggerated creates Earthy, Glamour, or Romantic auras and needs to be toned down when you're wearing your Classic Face.

Texture

Classic hair is clean, smooth, healthy, shiny, tidy.

Length

Hair touching or reaching below the shoulders does not actively present a classic image. It should be cut short, medium, or to swing slightly above the shoulders. Long hair is worn up for Classic Image.

Extremely long hair, falling to the shoulders or below, can be worn successfully with your Classic Face only if it is perfectly straight, and then only if you wish to present a down-to-earth or a sultry sort of Classic. To get the most out of your Classic Image, pin or tie down your very long hair into an upswept style.

Extremely short-cropped haircuts will not usually be successful conveyors of the Classic Image. Very short precision cuts, razor cuts, and "Sassoon" cuts produce Glamour and Earthy styles; if you wear Classic Face with them, you won't make a truly Classic statement. But at least they're more controlled and tidy than manes!

General Design

Hair design lines, cut shoulder-length and above, should be well-cut with clean lines. Clearly cut, sleek, vertical-line haircuts are most Classic: blunt cuts, straight hair, and medium-length cuts are ideal. Some Classic alternatives and variations are suggested on the following page. The silhouette should be as simple, unfussy, and symmetrically balanced as possible.

Classic Hair Variations

Parts

A side part, or no part, is Classic. Center parts are not; you may use a center focal point with no part instead of a center part. A part as little as a half-inch to either the left or the right side of center gives a more classic look.

Only a woman with precision-perfect, straight, symmetrical features, a receding chin, or a slightly round face should ever consider parting her hair in the center. And then only if she wishes to project an image other than Classic. If you wish to part your hair, part it at the side of your face.

Curls

Curls should not be kinky, frizzy, or fuzzy. The best curls are fat, smooth, and shiny (body waves or medium perms). The exception is that curls may be tight in afros on black women, which are Classic. Curls are of even and symmetrical length, cut well above the shoulders to frame the face. It is best to use hair spray or a permanent for uniformity and to prevent tousling.

Except for medium-length afros for black women, very curly hair tends to project either Earthy or Glamour Image, unless it is very carefully cut so that at least one variation is classically symmetrical, controlled, and elegant in feeling. The silhouette of the style should be smooth, even, and very tidy.

Waves

Natural, soft waves around the face are wonderful. Waves on the sides of the forehead and face are especially flattering when hair is upswept, or short and thick. They create an understatedly Classic Image.

Upswept

Any hairstyle worn upswept from the nape of the neck, especially if the design has soft waves that frame the face, can project the ultimate in classic feeling, so long as it isn't heavily "teased" into a "bouffant" (Glamour) style, or garnished with too many guiches, tendrils, or curls (Romantic or Glamour). Try moderate hair rolls, chignons, knots, and back twists.

Bangs

Absolutely straight, down-styled, full bangs are always classic in feeling; wispy or curly bangs are not. (Bangs rarely flatter the mature.)

Hair Colorings

Obviously dyed hair generally projects a Glamour look. If Classic Image is your primary choice and you wish to change your hair color, just remember that the more understated the change—the closer to your natural coloring—the better you'll project the Classic message. Check into "Colorful Confessions," the special section in this book on hair coloring, for further detail.

Hair Ornaments

Hairbands and Barrettes

Narrow hairbands and barrettes usually project a classic look. Promoting tidiness, they are functional and traditional rather than "high-fashion" fads. All these attributes are hallmarks of the clean lines, realism, and moderation exemplified by the true Classic.

They should be made of traditional materials like tortoise shell, horn, metal, cotton, grosgrain, and ivory. They are especially clever for those under thirty when monogrammed or hand-painted with town-and-country images such as ducks, geese, or garden flowers.

Be careful: no ornament for the Classic Image is flamboyant or competes for attention with any other facet of the appearance. "Unity is harmony" might well be the motto of the Classic. Ribbons, flowers, and glitter project Romantic and Glamour; scarves and athletic forehead bands project Earthy.

Combs

Hair combs, used to keep upswept hair tidy or to pull shoulder-length blunt-cuts up or back, may project Classic, if they are made of traditional materials, unobtrusive and not "high-fashion."

Accessorize Your Classic Face

Earrings
- Should not dangle or hang
- Should be between 1/4-inch and 1-inch in diameter
- No hoops, unless they're small, wide, expensive-looking, and worn with classic casual clothes. Even then they detract from your truly Classic Image.
- Best shape: circular, square, oval, button, love-knot, other knots that are knotted in 1/2-inch to 1-inch diameter. (Medium-sized rectangle or shell shapes may be appropriate for Classic if they fit the other criteria).
- Best materials: Florentine (brushed) metals, twisted or mixed metals (never highly shiny), pearl, ivory, gemstones other than diamond, plastic (though no clear, angular acrylics), tortoise shell, or any of these if antique; metal, hand-crafted, or stone beads, especially when smooth and oval.

Scarves

Scarves may be worn at the throat. When worn elsewhere—in the hair or at the waist—they usually project images other than Classic. Triangle-tied—worn front or to the side—is a favorite style. Add a silk tie for a bow at your blouse collar for a perennially Classic favorite.

Necklines and Collars

Man-tailored, notched lapel, and button-down collars are all instantly recognized as Classic. Stock collars and built-in ties are the ultimate in Classic. Peter Pan collars, boat-necks, and crew-necks are usually Classic.

Some Favorite Fabrics

Cotton broadcloth, tweed, angora, wool flannel, linen, wool, cotton, cotton/polyester, cashmere, silk, acrylic, oxford cloth, and flannel are all-time favorites.

Special Accessories
- Mock "horn-rimmed" glasses, and tortoise-shell rims
- Bow ties (floppy silk, collegiate men's, etc.)
- Argyle sweaters and socks
- Loafers, walking shoes, pumps, and other conservative leather shoes and medium-sized bags
- Shetland sweaters and wool plaid kilts
- Add-a-bead necklaces, leather watchbands

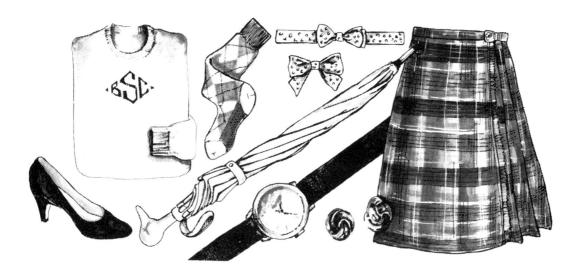

Classic Magic by Candlelight

You can add glow to your Classic Face for evening with touches of pink makeup and pearl powder. And a few more coats of mascara won't interfere with the balance of power in you features in the evening light, if you just barely stroke a bit more brow color on the arch of your classic brow.

If you'd like to give your eyes a hint of mystery and yet retain the Classic low-key eye makeup, subtly blend smoky grey, silver, or charcoal in the crease between top eyelid and underbrow bone. Careful—not too much, or you'll tip the balance of power away from the triangle of eyebrows, cheekbones, and lips. Keep the eyelids light and the brows stronger than the eyes.

Turn to the Candlelight Basics section in the back of the book to learn the basics of your extra pink and pearl touches, as well as other tips that can apply to your Classic evening look. Enjoy your glowing elegance, knowing that you are still understated, but not unstated by any means!

My Classic Model Face

What Do I Need to Know Before I Begin?

Use any technique that works for you in achieving the flawless complexion that so enhances the Classic Look. Also, don't forget that makeup is more beautifully blended when you use cremes with creme products, and then follow with the powder products.

Since you want to end with a matte finish, be sure to use sponges to apply your makeup on a clean pH-balanced (acidic) skin. The boundaries of the makeup you apply should never be noticeable in Classic.

Foundation should be one or two shades lighter than your skin tones and as "cool" as possible—not warm, sunny, honey, golden, tan, bronzy or peachy. Ivory, bisque, rachelle, sand, natural, oyster, ecru and light beige tones are all ideal.

The fairer you appear, the more translucent, clear, and perfect your skin will look. Keep your foundation-application touch light. Use very little, and blend it with those sponges. A heavy-handed "masque" of makeup doesn't create a Classic look—Glamour, maybe, but not Classic.

Crepey, mature, or unhealthy skin—from medication, sunbathing, or poor diet, for example—requires more **underbase tint and/or concealer,** less foundation, and a color more closely matching your natural skin tones.

Highlighter and concealer products are vital to the Classic Image. Choose the whitest and lightest concealers and highlighters (in your own best color range, of course). Reduce the "raccoon eyes" look by applying a light concealer under the eye in the inner (nose) half of the circle and a darker color on the outer half.

A little shimmer in your highlighter may be beautiful, but don't get carried away with iridescent ones; they leave the impression of Glamorous rather than Classic beauty.

Translucent Powder should always finish your ideal Classic complexion, again in the lightest color that becomes you. In addition to "setting" the foundation to stay and producing the appearance of poreless, matte finish, your powder helps keep the complexion oil-free, so the base doesn't darken, change color, or turn shiny.

If you use a very sheer layer of foundation, or none at all, you can get away with as much loose powder as you like to create that flawless Classic complexion look. More powder means a longer-lasting "face," too!

You can even top it all with a whisper of light pressed powder from a compact, for extra matte to your finish. And compacts are great to keep in your purse for touch-ups on an oily shine later. Remember, shiny isn't Classic.

Powder **Puff** Caution: Powder compact pads or "puffs" accumulate bacteria and oil when they are re-used. Change the soiled pad in your compact regularly (less often if it is a light powder used exclusively around the eyes). How? Purchase several loose ones, and keep them clean by rinsing them with an organic cleaner and/or hot water and allowing them to air-dry.

Be sure to dust under your eyes and the upper centers of your eyelids with powder to "set" white concealer creme in these areas (Light-colored top-eyelid centers are highly Classic.)

Eyebrow powders look even better when you also wear **eyebrow pencil** as instructed in this section. The eyebrow powder produces the look of a naturally full brow, and the pencil produces a well-defined, sharper brow. Be careful not to put on so much that your brows look artificial. Better to start with less and add more if you think you need it.

Classic Brows are meticulously groomed and arched. If you wear a Classic Face more than any other, you'll need to tweeze (or use cuticle scissors) a classic brow and arch for yourself. Keep in mind:

Thinner eyebrows adapt best to Romantic and Glamour Faces. Thin brows can always be thickened with cosmetics. Any obvious stray hairs on the orbital bone under the eyebrow should be tweezed or trimmed with cuticle scissors.

Thicker eyebrows adapt best to Earthy and some Glamour Faces. If your eyebrows are coarse, thick, or wiry, spray your eyebrow brush with hairspray, or use setting gel in that brush, and brush your brows to encourage the hairs to stay in place. Prune the most rebellious, for a Classic brow.

If you would like to keep your brows thicker and straighter because Earthy is the face you most often wear, just brush your brows into a classic arch and use brow powder—or better yet, pencil—to color a small triangle at the highest point of your arch, creating the illusion of a classic arch.

If you also remove the dozen or so most obvious hairs on the underside of your thick brow, you won't lose your Earthy Face, and your brows can then go either way. (Lighten them visually with a little face powder, if you like.)

Powder blushers were made for Classic. They're a super substitute for contour products, which are seldom subtle. Use them to add matte color and to softly define angles, especially the cheekbones. Keep the colors understated and the shimmer to a minimum.

Lips. Concentrate on making the two halves of your lips—from the center points, out toward the outer corners of the lips—appear as matched, mirror-twin images. Clara Bow pouts or sensuous Sophia Loren contours don't project the Classic Face very easily. If your lips are naturally too full, cover the outside line with a little concealer, under-base tint, foundation, or powder before you start.

Generally, your lips should be made up last, simply because it's easier to apply eye makeup without having to worry about smudging moist lip cosmetics with your palm.

To get a feeling for the Classic Face, the first few times you apply it, add your lip coloring first and then carefully apply eye makeup afterward so that it is less obvious than your lips. Once you're accustomed to the reduced amount of eye makeup worn in Classic Face, go back to the usual order of makeup application: eyes first, then lips.

Lipstick and lip makeup are opaque, medium-intensity colors in Classic Face. Enhanced lips need to dominate your eyes, and yet be just as prominent as eyebrows and cheekbones.

Light, clear glosses and pale frosted shades do not best project this image, but a medium color with a light hint of frost can be worn. For occasions when you really need to impress, stick to opaque, non-shiny shades. Pale frosteds or very, very dark or light shades project the other images. Don't even experiment with them for Classic.

Heavily-glossed lips are wonderful for Glamour or after-5:00 looks, but adding a heavy gloss diminishes the Classic appearance, unless your skin is extremely pale or your lips are extremely narrow and thin.

Lipliner used in shaping the lips gives them a well-defined, sculpted look in balance with the well-defined, sculpted cheekbones and eyebrows of the Classic Face. Don't go outside the natural lip line or let attention-seeking lipliner peep out unless you are correcting a flaw. Exaggeratedly exotic lips are more suited to your Glamour Face.

The creamier—and warmer-colored (less blue-based)—your lipliner pencil or product, the better it will hold lipstick within the lip line and maintain its perfection.

Since classical perfection of skin, and symmetry of feature, are the key factors in creating your Classic Face, you could technically stop right here.

But you may like a hint of **eye makeup**—to better define pale eye areas, to correct uneven skin tones around the eye, or to further build the impression of color that you're creating with your own natural eye color, hair, clothes, and other makeup. Keep eye shadow in the crease between eyelid and brow bone unless you have special contouring requirements.

If you are one of those fair ladies with pale features—such as light eyelashes, brows, and eyes—you may hate to leave the house without eye makeup because you feel the need to compensate for your lack of the dark drama so popular during the last few decades.

Actually, such medievally lovely ladies usually look best in Classic or Romantic Images, which do not harmonize with heavy eye makeup. Dark eye makeup tends to look stark if not downright overdone on such fair lilies and makes the rest of their features and their overall appearance seem washed out by comparison.

The less made-up, more subtle eyes of Classic and Romantic can give these women a delicate beauty and an overall glow that more than compensates for the absence of dark, dramatic eyes. Of course, very dimly lit restaurants can fade this gentle beauty, so a little more eye makeup in such lighting is called for.

Try an **eye makeup prep.** Apply a tiny bit of moisturizer to the skin under the eyes and the upper eyelids. After it has been blotted in/absorbed by the skin (and any excess wiped off), apply concealer and cover-up for the even skin tone look so desireable in Classic Face. Blot, and wipe off any remaining excess if necessary.

Then lightly apply a lighter-than-face-tone complexion powder (powder compact preferred to loose powder) to set the moisturizer and makeup, to aid in preventing makeup from smudging and running, and to further enhance the classic look of perfect skin and neutral color on the upper eyelids.

Eye makeup should not make your eyes more noticeable than the eyebrow, cheekbone, and lip triangle to retain your classic look. The best eye makeup treatment keeps eye shadows horizontal, opaque, subdued, and the eyelids light in color with minimal or no shimmer. Bulging eyes and prominent eyelids are the exception. They need slightly darker colors and barely-there liners to make the eye smaller and less dominating, in keeping with the classic triangle.

Eyeliner is seldom needed. If you feel you must use it, "don't let us see it" is the rule. Keep it to a hint: blurry, narrow, smoky, and smudged. Liquid liners must be lighter in color than your brows, kept thin and, if possible, in the lash-line itself. Use a cotton swab, the corner of your makeup sponge, or a fine-tip brush to blur the lines just before they dry. You might try dotting the skin between the lashes instead of drawing a line.

The more neutral **mascaras** project a classic feeling. A coat of pastel or colored mascara can be used over the basic neutrals if it suits your style and coloring. But keep in mind that striking, dramatic, not-found-in-nature colors don't create Classic as well as they do some of the other images.

Use a mascara comb (or brush), an eyebrow brush, or an old, dry mascara brush to separate lashes after applying mascara. Classic Face lashes should look natural and not heavily coated.

A word of caution: less mascara is best when extra moisturizer and creamy highlighter are applied. Why? The extra moisture will tend to smudge mascara onto the skin around the eyes, unless the mascara is extremely waterproof. Keep in mind that super-waterproof mascara tends to be harsh on lashes.

If you choose to use **artificial eyelashes** for evening Classic wear, use the individual type, still keeping eye shadow color to a minimum, and use short lashes, applied so that they're undetectable. Only deep-set eyes can really carry off artificial lashes successfully in the Classic Image.

On the following pages is a chart of the step-by-step techniques to use in creating the Model Classic Face. They are not hard, and once you're familiar with them, you can work faster and they don't take a whole lot longer than the Fast Face. You will be thrilled with the perfection that is your result!

Classic Model Face: Tool Checklist

Cosmetic Products

☐ Under-base tint, or pre-makeup
☐ Light Concealer (and possibly medium-color too)
☐ Foundation/Makeup Base:
   —lightest possible color
   —Ivory/Beige/or Bisque preferred
☐ Highligher:
   —opaque, minimal shimmer, light color
☐ Translucent Powder (light color, and non-shimmer)
☐ Eyebrow Pencil
☐ Eyebrow Powder:
   —dry cake brush-on, with stiff brush
☐ Creme Rouge:
   —medium color
   —opaque, minimal shimmer
☐ Powder Blush: (non-shimmer)
   —dark, for hollowing and gentle facial contour
   —possibly a lighter one as well, for eye shadow
☐ Lipliner:
   —the warmest color in your color key
   —pencil preferred
☐ Lipstick:
   —medium-color
   —opaque, or with a mere hint of frost
☐ Optional: Medium-color Eye Shadow, Mascara,
            Light-color Pressed Powder, White Pencil

Cosmetic Tools

☐ Makeup "silk" sponge
☐ Powder complexion brush and powder pad
☐ Natural sea sponge
☐ Eyebrow brush
☐ Lipstick brush
☐ Mascara comb and eye shadow brush

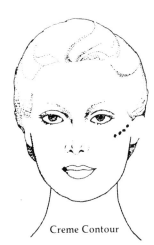

Complexion

Model Face—Classic Formula

Complexion, Eyebrow, Cheekbone, Lip

1. Classic Complexion

Thinly smooth on under-base tint with sponge, to level and color-correct.

Generously dab concealer onto blemishes, veins, liver spots, under-eye shadows, and any other flaws. Pat very lightly to soften "edges."

Contour with any other creme contour products you want to use to sculpt or correct the face via lights and shadows.

Take a look in the special Contouring section of this book for more detail.

Spread your foundation sparingly with a makeup sponge, avoiding eye and lip areas unless contouring. The correct color won't need to reach to the hairline.

Creme Contour

2. Classic Cheekbones

Dot creme rouge along the cheekbone itself, starting somewhere below the outer third of the eye, and ending toward the temple hairline. Blend with sponge.

Dust translucent powder onto the greater cheekbone area, to "set" the cremes.

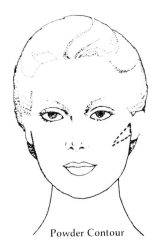

Powder Contour

With powder blusher, hollow out the underside of the cheekbone, drawing the blusher from about mid-ear level toward the lip, in the natural hollow under the cheekbone.

The closer you bring it to the outside corner of your mouth, the more you sculpt the cheekbones.

Powder Blusher Cautions: *too heavy a layer isn't Classic, and *don't bring the blusher any closer to the nose than the center of the face (the center of the face is directly below the pupil of the eye when you're looking straight ahead into the mirror). Closer to the nose produces a Romantic, not Classic, look, and very close broadens the nose.

3. Complexion Finishing, for a Matte Finish

Pour loose powder into the powder pad. Fold the pad in half, with the powder on the inside. Then rub the two sides of the pad together so that the powder is ground into the pad and is not loose on its surface. Pat the face with the pad, several times, including under-eyes and eyelid centers.

Next, sprinkle some loose powder into its jar cap, and dust a little with your brush over any areas of generously applied concealer or too-creamy products. Brush off any excess powder that collects loosely in dry patches.

If you're left a bit dusty or dry, or if powder has clumped in areas, dampen a natural sea sponge, wring it "dry" in a towel, lightly pat it over the dry areas.

This step "sets" the makeup allowing it to last longer during your day. It restores the look and feel of natural (moist) skin without removing the desired perfect, matte finish.

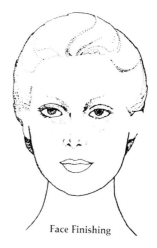

Face Finishing

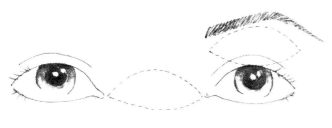

Ideal Eye

4. Classic Eyebrows

Here is the ideal eye. Decide where your eyebrow should begin. If your eyes are too close together, start the brows farther apart. If your eyes are too far apart, try bringing your brow makeup a little closer to the nose than the ideal start-point, which is directly over the tear duct.

Arch the brow with eyebrow powder and with or without eyebrow pencil. By looking straight ahead into the mirror, you can determine the spot for the highest point of the brow (the arch)—it will be above the colorful iris of the eyeball, to the iris's outside rim (the side toward the ear).

(See Contour section for additional detail).

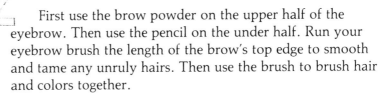

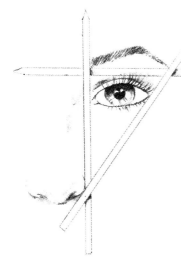

First use the brow powder on the upper half of the eyebrow. Then use the pencil on the under half. Run your eyebrow brush the length of the brow's top edge to smooth and tame any unruly hairs. Then use the brush to brush hair and colors together.

Eyebrow Contouring with Lights

Now is the time to use your creme, pencil, and powder contour products to highlight your eyebrow area.

On top of your moisturizer, you may use a very sheer, creamy, moist highlighter on the crowsfeet and fine lines at the outer corner of the eyes, to help soften the lines visually. Often—with time and nourishing products—these lines may soften permanently.

Try this easy olive-fork method of highlighting the brow, outer-eye, and upper cheekbone area with highlighter to emphasize your now angular cheekbones and dominant eyebrows.

With your white pencil or highlighter powder, draw a line just underneath the brow. (If you used pencil, you might now repeat on top of it with a highlighter powder, to set and enhance.) Line near the brow from the highest point of the arch out toward the temple.

To finish, brush the highlighter powder to travel parallel above your creme rouge on the cheekbone, the length of the cheekbone, to the temple. Also, dust your jawline to "square" it for this image, if needed. Blur the contour "edges" lightly with makeup sponge.

Classic Brows Arch

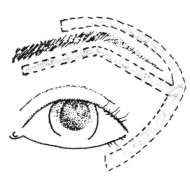

Olive-Fork Highlighting

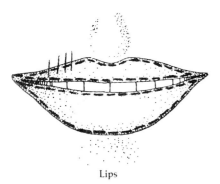

Lips

5. Classic Lip

Cover lip edges with powder, foundation, or concealer, if you haven't already.

Just inside the lip line, use lipliner to outline the lips to create a look of perfectly symmetrical, well-defined lips.

Apply medium-color, opaque lipstick with a lip brush for a long-lasting precision look. Do not add gloss.

6. Classic Eye Makeup

Choose a horizontal eye makeup technique that leaves the underbrow and eyelid as light as possible. The crease (between top lid and bone) may be emphasized. Blend edges.

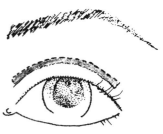
Crease Emphasis

Top eyelid's center should be light to white. Use cream concealer or highlighter. Pat with light powder, powder highlighter, or lightest shadow. (If cream concealer isn't used, use highlighter powder or light powder on the eyelid center.)

Keep eyeliner to a minimum, if used at all, and on the outer third of the top and bottom eyelids, close to lashes. Blur it.

Curled lashes draw attention to your Classic highlighted brow bone, if eye shadow is light and the area between brow and crease is light.

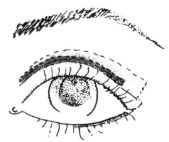
Horizontal Eye Makeup

Apply mascara thinly, and comb or brush out afterward.

Keep all eye color under the umbrella of the eyebrow. Any dark shadow is in the crease (between top eyelid and bone) or wrapped around the outside corner of the eye (outer third, only, of top/bottom lids).

Don't exaggerate eye color up and out toward the hairline unless necessary for critical contour correction.

7. Classic Wrap-Up

Final whisk of pressed (or loose) powder pad, for extra poreless look, to merge any remaining blusher "edges," and as anti-shine.

Review the Check-Out earlier in this Classic chapter to be sure your final product follows the Classic Face formula. And congratulations on a job well done!

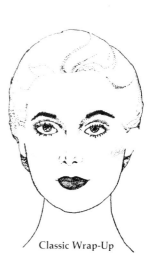
Classic Wrap-Up

The Classic Image for the Career Woman

The Classic aura is made for you and your success! If you want to look healthy, wealthy, and wise, and to project a success or authority image to gain respect in the workplace—you've just found your guaranteed business style.

As any successful advertising or image agency will tell you, initially it's not necessarily how well a product works that makes it sell. It's how well it appears that the product will work.

Psychological studies have shown for years that employers, employees, and clients still make instant decisions based on appearance marketability—on image! You do it too! You judge the taste, confidence, sense, capability, and effectiveness of others in a matter of seconds, before you even hear a word spoken.

It's fruitless to protest that you're capable, or that your product is good. The fact is that in a first impression, others judge you by what you seem to be. They may never get to know the real you if you don't make a success of that first impression!

Your professional image can open doors. A factor that companies consider when they promote their key personnel is their capacity to project success images. Don't set yourself up for reduced success by failing to take advantage of the extra edge that appropriate image-projection can achieve for you.

Once your success image is securely in place, those talents you've now wrapped in the Classic Image will emerge and carry you to the top. Maintaining the Classic Image thereafter supports the impression that you're doing a good job. Should you choose to wear one of the other three images to the office, you'd lose the reliable image you've gained.

Professional Image: Makeup and Apparel

Before you choose makeup and apparel colors, consider your type of office lighting.

If you are a lucky one who works in natural light or in incandescent—(standard light bulb)—light, almost all of the colors appropriate to a professional environment will be flattering.

But be careful if your natural coloring is cool. Clear, cool coloring ("*Winter/Contrast/Sunrise*") looks a bit too warm and yellow in standard-bulb light. You need to choose the most vivid or "warmest" colors from your cool range, so that you don't clash with the lighting. The same can be said for mild and cloudy, cool coloring (*"Summer/Gentle/Sunlight"*). You need to choose your "warmest" (you don't have many vivid shades) colors from your cool range, too.

More likely, you work in the fluorescent lighting that is currently prevalent. It throws an ashy, greenish cast onto the skin. If your natural coloring is warm and clouded (*"Autumn/Muted/Sunset"*), then you're in luck. Everyone else tends to look sallow, muddy-skinned, washed out, or merely green. Pink and purple colors flatter no one in fluorescent light.

If your natural coloring is cool, wear your cool colors but choose the warmest of them for fluorescent light. For example, if your coloring is clear and cool (*"Winter/Contrast/Sunrise"*), your true reds look better than your bright burgundy. (Remember no purple? Burgundy leans to purple.) Red is just one of your warmer colors. For example, a hot, almost-black navy, or a vivid royal blue will flatter more than your icy shades. All your colors look good under standard bulbs.

If your coloring is mild and softly cool (*"Summer/Gentle/Sunlight"*), choose a night-light red or warm berry in your cool key for fluorescent light. Or choose one of your least steely blue-greys, or a soft off-white.

If you have a mild, clear kind of warm coloring (*"Spring/Light-Bright/Sunlight"*), you can look bronze and ashy—the opposite of your clear appeal—in fluorescent lighting. In addition to keeping artificial hair blonding to a minimum (it turns very green), compensate by wearing your hottest, clearest colors such as flame, light orange, and French vanilla. Try to stand under incandescent light whenever you get the opportunity. It is the most flattering to your kind of coloring.

Choose your office cosmetics with care. Although some sparkle can be worn with the evening Classic Face, your business-like Classic is best achieved with opaque, non-shiny products—a must for your professional life.

Nail polish, lipstick, and eye shadow should all be matte and opaque. Powder blush cannot be iridescent and should have as little frost as possible. Translucent powder is one of your most important tools for an overall matte finish and to achieve a face that lasts.

Contouring should not be done with browns in flourescent lighting, since it turns "muddy" under that light and you tend to look like a road map with lines of color everywhere!

Be sure to follow the instructions for Classic eye makeup prep in the Model Face instructions. This will help prevent black under-eyes while you're concentrating on the professional task at hand and haven't time for frequent touch-ups.

Eye makeup colors closest to neutral and natural tones project the most polished office image. This is true for shadows, eyeliners, and mascara. Do not wear dramatic, glamour makeup, or use glamour techniques, for the office. Leave false eyelashes, trendy colors, pale lips, sultry-kohl eyeliners, and bright, faddish color mascaras, lipsticks, and nail polishes for other images and occasions.

Nail polishes that are not man-made colors, including those close to the natural color of the nails or skin, are good choices. People watch your hands when you talk, so keep your nails manicured.

The clear, natural red polishes are the best reds. Be careful—reds often rub off on papers, leaving an unprofessional trail behind.

Professional Image: Hair

Tailored, controlled, hairstyles win the day by presenting the most powerful professional success image. Since most of us do not have perfectly trouble—free hair, it's probably a subliminal message: "If she can control her hair, she can probably control any situation!"

Women with silver-grey hair or brunette have a psychological advantage in the business world, especially if they have cool coloring (*"Winter/Contrast/Sunrise*, and *Summer/Gentle/Sunlight"*). Hair color close to your own natural color projects the conservative-yet-dynamic impression that takes you far in the business world. See the special section in this book, "Colorful Confessions," for more information on hair coloring and the career woman (including more on the influence of fluorescent lights on altered hair color).

The Professional Woman vs. Fashion Fads

Trend-setting styles in makeup, jewelry, hair, and apparel are fun for off-hours images. They make a pleasant change when your office day has ended. They are not appropriate and do not benefit you in the professional setting.

Fad colors tend to be unnatural colors, unflattering in fluorescent lighting and not Classic/Professional. They are also impractical purchases for business makeup and clothing, which are usually selected for timeless appeal and wearability, quality, and investment. (If we were rich enough to invest in short-use expensive clothes, we'd probably be doing something else!)

There is an exception! If you are in a field where a slightly glamorous style is widely accepted because it builds that enterprise's image (the arts, for instance), then you may wear the strongest Classic statement that you can create, stretching the Classic guidelines for medium colors and styles a little.

It's better not to tamper with the Classic Face formula, however, because any deviation from it keeps it from happening! But an haute couture blouse, a scarf tied with more than the usual flair, earrings a little more dramatic than regular Classic, and your strongest Classic colors can add drama in a work environment requiring high-fashion professionalism.

If you decide that's not enough drama, then turn to the Glamour Face and follow it completely—with no mixing in of the Classic Face—but as conservatively as you like. Just be aware that Glamour Image makes another statement entirely, and consider your professional position. The higher up the rung, the more you can relax your conservative look. No matter how high you've advanced, Classic can be counted on when you've got to be sure.

Chapter 2

The Earthy Face

Setting the Mood

If you're ready for a flattering image that is totally natural, then here's the look for you! Easy to pull together and easy to wear, your Earthy Image has you ready for anything. And that's good, because your earthy personality is always ready for new experiences. Earthy Image projects your fun-loving side. The Earthy look may give you a sensual or carefree appearance.

Characterized by its lack of conformity, the close-to-nature feelings evoked by an Earthy statement can give life to your free spirit, allowing you to step out of traditional roles into freedom.

Enjoy your "flaws" as well as your assets. Earthy Image can capitalize on them, turning them into interesting individuality. Leave responsibilities behind when you call forth this face. (Isn't that an irresistible lure?)

How Did Earthy Image Become So Popular?

Women for centuries have loved expressing their sensuality with exotic Earthy. In cultures where "civilization" and "high-tech" are not governing ideals, women have captured the essence of Earthy's freedom.

Armed with natural cosmetics like henna and kohl, fibers like gauze and leather, and objets d'art from shells to fur, these women have woven a beauty image that revels in the senses. Earthy unself-consciously enjoys its overt, physical origins and siren suggestiveness.

The closer your face, hair and garments are to the original inspiration, the more powerful your Earthy message will be to other people.

Tone down your texture and color volume slightly, and your Earthy Image becomes either saucily impish, or carefree, California natural, perfect with (even if not forever in) blue jeans. As the return-to-nature movement grew in the 1960's, the wholesome beauty of day-at-the-beach freshness—long, loose hair, tousled and sun-streaked, and freshly-scrubbed faces—left its geographic boundaries to solidly enter the ranks of contemporary beauty imagery.

Famous Earthy Faces

Although the earthy look was dramatized by Bizet's time-tested and popular "Carmen," Hollywood didn't unreservedly endorse Earthy until the 60's and 70's. Then every nuance of this image began to be employed by actresses like sloe-eyed Sophia Loren, dramatic young Jane Fonda, and casual Goldie Hawn.

Ava Gardner, Raquel Welch, Jacqueline Bisset, Julie Christie, Brooke Shields, and of course Sophia prefer a duskier, more sensual Earthy than the California—natural types like Farrah Fawcett, Candice Bergen, Bo Derek, Yoko Ono, and Cheryl Tiegs. Ali McGraw and Mariel Hemingway are somewhere in between.

Why and When Do You Wear Earthy Image?

You choose Earthy Image when you're feeling either very casual, or sensual. Think gypsy, native, artistic, sporty, jungle, feline, foxy, wild tigress, nautical, athletic, western, bohemian, organic, professorial, scientific, wanderer—for a few!—when you choose this face. Relaxed and suntanned have greater affinity for this image than almost any other mood.

Earthy presents such a wholesome message that it's a natural for sport clothes and athletic gear. It spells "healthy and alive."

No other image shows off your tan or complements the relaxed resort aura as well as this sun-kissed face. For your beach-combing vacations, pop your Earthy kit in your bag with your bathing suit. Or maybe you'd just like that sun-drenched look, since you haven't had a vacation lately.

Are you in the mood to wear a loose-fitting Greek import, or do you just want out of your conservative suit? Put on your Earthy Face. Go on safari in your own back yard, to the Greek Isles while marketing, or to Mexico at dinner. This look is a vagabond wanderer's delight.

Perhaps you're looking for a more dramatic response from others? You need to pass for a young and struggling college student, or someone who hasn't yet acquired serious worries? Or more radically still, you need a strong non-conformist, non-materialistic image? You can make each of those statements in your Earthy style.

Earthy is effective when you want to make men realize your blatant temptress appeal and interest without having to resort to overtly glamorous tactics that may strike a false note for you. Pick up your kohl stick and try your exotic Earthy for effect. And does it have effect!

Perhaps sultry or sunny are not quite your mood? There's also saucy elfin, urchin, spritely, impish, or gamin to project with Earthy, especially when your hair is short. You need only add the merest hint of makeup, using the Earthy formula, to capture such whimsy.

Earthy Image: For the excitingly "natural" you.

Where Do You Wear Your Earthy Face?

As a runner—or non-runner who wears running gear—you'll love this face. Anytime you're playing active sports which make even your face perspire, you won't want the makeup running off with the plays. Score points with your Earthy Face, instead.

Clamdigging, fishing, boating, cookouts, hiking, hunting, skiing, climbing, riding dirt bikes, camping and similar open-air activities were made for Earthy. It's the natural face for sunny beaches and poolside tanning, so bring your Earthy tools along with your towels and suntan lotion.

When you're dining in an ethnic restaurant, and are dressed for the theme, pull it all together with the most appropriate face: Earthy. Whether the food is Tex-Mex western, urban cowboy, Indian, Greek, Scandinavian, Italian, Roman, Middle Eastern, Mexican, French, or South American, your Earthy aura will make both you and the face more intriguing.

If you're trying to teach, paint, write, or need an arty or artistic look, here's the ideal face.

What are the Characteristics of the Earthy Face?

Gauguin, Picasso, and Rembrandt all loved to paint the Earthy woman. She is eternally fascinating, warm, sensual. Her eyes draw you, and have always been her greatest point of emphasis.

The Earthy Face is characterized by vibrant and warm skin, and dominant eyebrows and eyes. Thick, straight brows sensuously attract, and dusky, sultry eyes demand attention.

If your mood is more carefree and casual than exotic, keep cosmetics to a lick and a promise, and sport your tan. To make your casual face reflect a sensual, duskier, more mysterious beauty, keep the same balance of power in the eyes and brows; just use a little more smoke and dust to dramatize the eyes.

The Formula—the easiest one around:

- healthy, glowing skin—preferably tanned or dusky
- the look of strong, compelling eyes and eyebrows
- medium-to-strong colors
- hair, and none of it need be tidy

If you've already got these attributes, you'll slide right in. If you're a bit of a pale lily, hide your hair brush for a day or two, slick gleamer or bronzer over your nose for a home-grown suntan, apply some gorgeous eye makeup, and you will cross home plate.

Introducing You to the Earthy Formula

Do I Have Time for It?

Feel like wearing no makeup at all? Then loosen your hair, step into a pair of jeans, and wash everything off your face (except the mascara if you're really pressed for time). In 60 seconds or less, you can look freshly scrubbed and glowingly casual.

Instead of stroking on an inappropriate lipstick and blusher, just dash on some lip gloss, and creme or liquid "sunshine" for face color. The same amount of time will have been spent, but with very different results.

The sun-kissed face will enhance your mood of freedom. Casual clothes worn with lipstick only look wrong and out of place—too studied and formal for your more casual mood. If you prefer a less casual look for your sporty hours, perhaps you'd be happier with tailored lines of clothes and Classic Face.

When you want stronger allure, a more decided statement, or a face to go with a man-trap garment, each minute you add to creating your face will only turn up its power of attraction.

Naturally-dusky skin types, and faces with strong brows, hardly need to lift a finger to put on this face. You don't need to be left out, however, if you're fair-skinned or have skinny brows. Just add a few more cosmetic items to your bag.

And speaking of ease, your hair requires as little effort as the face. Loose, long, untamed, unruly hair feels great and looks better when Earthy is to be your statement. Youthful sun-worshippers and outdoor enthusiasts will especially appreciate cultivating this image for its speed, convenience, and flexibility.

Does Earthy Image Work For Me?

If your skin is healthy and you're comfortable with the look of little to no makeup, you can wear a wholesome sunny face. If not, try the sultrier Earthy, which can carry a heavier makeup.

Since a tan, or the look of one, can make your carefree look work, this may not be your favorite face in the dead of winter (if you become pale then). But if you're one of the lucky—healthy, sultry-skinned rain or shine—this face will work for you year-round.

If you'd rather turn up the suggestiveness than have quite such a shower-clean feeling, cosmetics can make this face work by warming pale complexions and making every woman's eyes an invitation. Dark brows and lashes aren't essential, but they do help. Full lips are nice, too (think of Sophia Loren, Raquel Welch).

Face Shapes: Any face shape will work. Inverted triangular (heart-shaped) faces look particularly sultry, since the width of the forehead and eye area add more dominance to the brows and eyes.

Coloring: Dusky skins adapt most readily to a toned-down, sun-kissed face. Pale skins really look best in Earthy with a tan or sun suggestion. Dusky skins and dark leashes also need less artifice to create a sensual aura, but everyone can find her most "come-hither" face.

Earth tones and natural colors are a must for this look. If you know that your strong coloring is *"Winter/Contrast/Sunrise"* or, even better, *"Autumn/Muted/Sunset,"* you probably won't be surprised to learn that it is easiest for you to achieve Earthy. You also tend to have the most natural drama in your coloring. (Don't lose heart, pale *"Summers* and *Springs,"* the makeup bag's not far away, and Earthy doesn't require that much of it.)

Skin Types: The entire range of skin types can wear Earthy Face. Suntans are, of course, ideal, as are naturally dusky skin tones. Blemish-free skin is more important than color. Freckles work with Earthy, especially with the carefree look. Beauty marks do well with the exotic Earthy mood. Skin tones should always be warm.

Ages: Carefree, casual Earthy is most attractive on the youthful. Dark circles and discoloration usually preclude the more mature woman's use of Earthy. Every age, except the very young, can step up the look and enjoy their most sultry face. The more exotic Earthy looks make very youthful faces look hard, however. Young ladies should be encouraged to enjoy carefree Earthy and turn up the power for dramatic Earthy only as they mature into women and look natural in it.

Eyebrows and Eyes: When you look at an Earthy Face, the eyes are the first feature you notice. The eyes and brows steal the show. Keep the lines for both features horizontal.

Strong, wild brows that demand attention by moving straight across the face make the most powerful and quickly identifiable statement. The thinner, more controlled the brow, the more diluted your Earthy message.

Lots of mascara on dark lashes are a key element. Don't curl your lashes, rather, encourage them to be straight and spiky. Eye makeup will vary from a merely dusting of the lids from lash to brow to the feline message of elongated, cat eyes.

Lips are not emphasized. They can be toned down with neutrals, or glossed. If they are full, or barely lined with neutral pencil, they make the sultry Earthy statement.

If your skin is warm and clear, your eyebrows dominant, untamed, and dark, your lips pale, and your eyes seductive, this may be the easiest face for you. You may only need face color, but if you're glowing from the sun, you may not even need that!

To summarize the basics for creating your Earthy Face:

- complexion - warm, clear
- eyebrows - straight, strong, unruly
- eyes - almond, elongated, attention-grabbing
- lips - no emphasis, gloss, perhaps pencil liner
- colors - sun-drenched, earth-tones, naturals, and jungle-dark colors

Earthy Fast Face

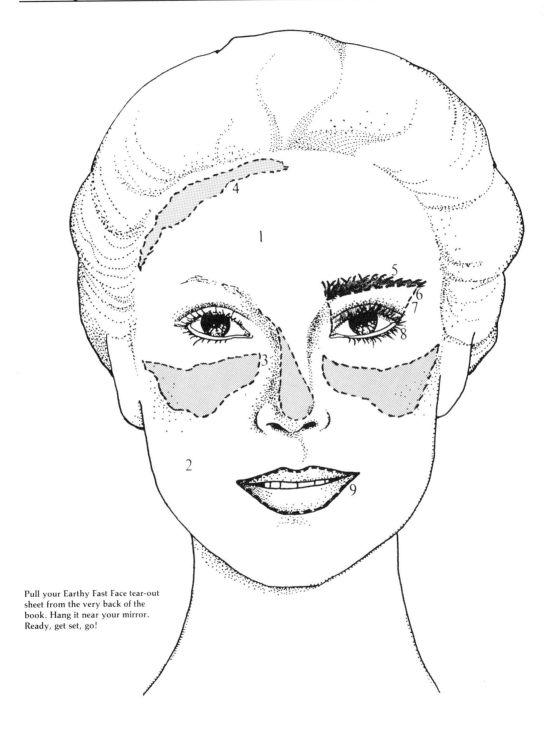

Pull your Earthy Fast Face tear-out
sheet from the very back of the
book. Hang it near your mirror.
Ready, get set, go!

Let your hair reflect your freedom—loose, unfettered, and easy-to-care-and-wear. This face is designed to complement down-to-earth dressing and Mother Nature's own accessories.

Even though Earthy appears to take little or no effort, there is an art to creating the Image. If you'll follow the formula carefully, you'll be pleasantly surprised at how much impact so simple a formula can have.

Ready Now for Your 8-Minute Makeover?

Regardless of whether you use Fast Face or Model Face, you will sport a delightful Earthy Face when you follow the easy formula. Just remember that emphasis on eyebrows and eyes is everything, and you'll be as magnetic as anyone!

—Fast Face—Earthy Formula

Eyebrow and Eye Emphasis, and Natural Face

Complexion

1 Do I need foundation? If so, just barely apply a warm color, with makeup sponge
2 Cover blemishes only—not freckles—with medium-tone concealer

Face Color

3 Copy the sun's kiss: cheek to cheek across the nose, using creme, gel, or liquid color
4 Lightly "sun kiss" either the temples or just above the eyebrow, or the forehead, nose and chin (your choice)

Eyebrows

5 Use brow brush to brush hairs straight up for an unruly appearance
6 Use brow powder to darken a straight line across the under-brow skin (to camouflage arch, and darken and thicken brow)

Eyes

7 Dust with smoky, earth-tone shadow from lash to brow
8 Mascara the lashes: little for carefree, more heavily for exotic

Lips

9 Touch with gloss for carefree, or line lip edges with neutral pencil for exotic

The Total Look

Pulling It All Together for Earthy Image

1. Natural, warm, tan, or dusky skin: appearance of little makeup. Medium-to-dark foundation color.
2. Upper half of the face dominates, especially eyebrows and eyes. Features are horizontally emphasized. Eyebrows are straight across face, and often unruly.
4. Eyes are sultry—slanted, almond, or elongated—lined, and shadowed from dusty to smoky. Area from lash to brow is shaded.
5. Cheek and face color is applied with the look of sun.
6. Lips are touched with gloss, or neutral lipliner pencil.
7. Colors are neutrals, earth tones, or dusty.

Eyebrows
1. Bold, dark, wide
2. Straight across
3. Unruly and wild

Complexion
1. Warm, dusky, sun-kissed
2. Natural

Cheekbones
1. Sun-kissed cheek color extends horizontally across face, nose
3. Little to no shine
4. Creme, gel, stick, or liquid color

Lips
1. Gloss or neutral pencil liner
2. No emphasis

Hair
1. Unruly, untamed, unfettered, wild, windblown, loose
2. No smooth, rounded lines
3. Straight braids, frizzy hair, or long, straight hair
4. Lion's mane long perms or layers
5. Center part, or hair brushed away from face to back of head
6. Brushed forward, then tossed back for volume

Eye Makeup
1. Horizontal, dusty to smoky
2. Wide, elongated, smoky eyeliner
3. Smoky, dusty colors; kohl
4. Darken area from brow to lash with shadow

Ornaments
1. Natural materials and textures like feathers, shells, etc.
2. Dangling, loose
3. Non-glitter

Garments
1. Sports and outdoor attire
2. Native, casual, loose, sensual, natural materials
3. Non-traditional, carefree, non-dramatic

Buzz Words
1. Sun-kissed, Carefree, Well-scrubbed, Wholesome
2. or Wild, Sensual, Dusky
3. Eyes and Eyebrows
4. Natural Materials, Fabrics
5. Natural Colors and Earth Tones
6. Neutrals
7. Nails: Clear, or Earth Tones
8. Fragrance: Light, casual, mellow, or musky, woodsy, primeval

Check It Out, and Go!

If I'm not tan or dusky, is my foundation too light? Does it conceal too much?

Are my eyebrows strong? Dark enough? Straight across?

Are my eyes as prominent as my brows? Are the lids darkened?

Does my face look like it's been touched by the sun?

Are my fingernails light-colored and medium length for my sunny mood, or long and earth-toned for my sultry?

Doesn't freedom to express your casual self feel great? Passing your checkout means you look as wonderful as you feel!

Earthy Color Palette

Colors of the earth warmed by the sun project an Earthy Image. They are medium to dark, and the "warmest" shades of your own coloring range.

If you are in the light-hearted Earthy mood, natural and light earth tones will speak your mind: salmon, honey, rust, camel, rosy beige, grayed navy, and strong yellow are some examples.

If you prefer to project exotic Earthy, darker and stronger colors will increase your mystique. Pick your shades from among intense earthy colors like cordovan, taupe, medium golden brown, medium yellow—green, gold, brown-black, charcoal blue-grey, and mahogany.

When you're choosing between a subdued or a bright version of a color, go for the most subdued, muted, cloudy shade that can still suit your coloring. The brighter your choice, the less mystique you convey, and Earthy is, after all, the misty mystery of Autumn or the sunset enigma of the desert at dusk. If you are wearing your warmest, darkest colors, you may add metallic shimmer to your makeup and clothes for sultry or evening Earthy image.

Have you guessed, then, that the color key most suited to the Earthy look is the yellow-based, ashy key (*Autumn/Muted/Sunset*)?

Think medium-to-dark, earth warmed by the sun, neutrals.

Some Suggested Colors

Dark dull red

Smoky grey

Grey

Grey-beige (cold taupe)

Light true green

True green

Black-brown

Dark Chinese blue

Buff and light clear gold

Light warm beige

Clear camel

Honey and light amber

Medium golden brown

Clear orange red

Medium or bright yellow green

Light salmon, apricot, orange or peach

Russets

Copper and rust-orange

All browns and yellow golds

Golden bronze

Terra cotta and brick

Burnt sienna, burnt umber

Dark salmon, peach, apricot

Moss green, olive green

Grey-greens, greige

Rosy brown

Rosy beige

Light pink cocoa, cool mocha

Cherrywood

Rosewood

Cordovan

Grey-blue

Greyed navy

Sample Makeup Color Schemes

Natural Red Scheme

Concealer: None, medium flesh tone, or dark

Foundation: "Sunniest" beige tone becoming to you—up to 3 shades darker than your natural skin tones

Face Powder: None, medium, or dark

Highlighter: None

Creme Rouge: Dusty red, brick, or sunny pink

Powder Blush: None

Lip Pencil: Bronzed, dull red

Lipstick: Lip gloss

Mascara: Clear black-brown

Eye Shadow: Smoky grey

Orange Coral Scheme

Concealer: None, or medium flesh tone

Foundation: Dark, warm peachy beige, up to 2 shades darker than your natural skin tones

Face Powder: None, medium, or dark

Highlighter: Honey or yellow

Creme Rouge: Bright orange or orange-coral

Powder Blush: Used as eye shadow: Orange coral or honey amber

Lip Pencil: Honey or light amber

Lipstick: Lip gloss

Mascara: Clear brown-black

Eye Shadow: Honey or clear warm amber

For the information of the serious color student:

Clear, Cold, Blue-based
(Winter/Contrast/Sunrise)

Clear, Warm, Yellow-based
(Spring/Light-Bright/Sunlight)

Sample Color Schemes

Dusty Mocha Scheme

Concealer: None, medium, or dark

Foundation: Cool beiges, or dark rachelles—up to 3 shades darker than your skin tones

Face Powder: None, medium, or dark

Highlighter: None

Creme Rouge: Mocha; dusty pink; rosewood

Powder Blush: None

Lip Pencil: Cocoa, cherrywood, mocha, rosy coffee

Lipstick: Lip gloss

Mascara: Greyed black

Eye Shadow: Slate, raisin, rosy brown

Terra Cotta Scheme

Concealer: None, medium or dark

Foundation: Warm, honey bronze, copper, tan or sunny tones up to 2 shades darker than your skin tones

Face Powder: None, medium, or dark

Highlighter: Dark earth shimmers—gold, bronze, ecru

Creme Rouge: Dusty rust, burnt orange, dusty honey, mahogany, terra cotta

Powder Blush: None

Lip Pencil: Burnt orange, rust, brown tones, salmon, dusty apricot

Lipstick: Lip gloss

Mascara: Brown

Eye Shadow: Moss, avocado, olive, bronze, gold, greige, greyed yellow-green, coffee, mustard

For the information of the serious color student:

Cloudy, Cool, Blue-based (Summer/Gentle/Sunlight)

Cloudy, Warm, Yellow-based (Autumn/Muted/Sunset)

Earthy Hair

Earthy is casual. The fun of dressing in down-to-earth style is in the ease with which you wear it—and that includes your Earthy hair. Thanks to great perms and cuts, women have made enormous progress in attractive hairstyles that are comfortable and trouble-free.

Don't strive to achieve elegance or symmetry—don't even pick up your blow dryer! Earthy Image is the only one where positively frizzy can be truly beautiful.

Straight braids, pigtails, and ponytails are as practical for your brisk activities as they are enhancers of your Earthy look.

Any length can be coaxed into its most capricious, free-form style, and most hairstyles straight from the shower will look carefree, especially permed hair and short or layered cuts. You might even want to try protein sculpture lotion to maintain that earthy wild look that wet hair achieves.

Texture

Think tousled, carefree, loose, casual, uncontrolled, kinky, layered, dangling, wild. Kinky perms look like a natural hairstyle; back-combing does not—that's Glamour. Look as if you just got out of bed; run your fingers through your hair or flip it. Looking as though you can go for a ride in a convertible without dismay only adds to your style—and style you've got! Just remember to keep it natural.

Length

Long hair, below the shoulders, is a natural for Earthy Image. Most shorter lengths will usually work, too, except for very carefully controlled or sleek styles, which belong to other moods.

Very, very short lengths worn wild or sculpted tend to project a glamour style but if you wear exceptionally heavy eyebrows and do not use sculpting lotion, you may be able to project a glamorous sort of earthy. This is tricky, and if you chose such a hairstyle, you were probably aiming for Glamour, anyway, so it may be best for you to turn to the Glamour chapter and create for yourself a sensual sort of Glamour, instead.

General Design

Haircut designs should be ignored or coaxed into the freest form. Blunt cuts on hair that has body, layered cuts, and straight hair are the easiest to work with. The only formal precision cut that always projects Earthy is the precision cut with a center part, which you blow dry straight back toward the center back of your head. Horizontal emphasis is better than vertical.

Hairstyles should be as natural as possible, and be angled away from the face, toward the back of the head whenever possible. Vent brushes help layer air and fluff into the hair. Volume is mandatory for an earthy look, unless you've opted for the elfin look of short hair.

Another volume technique is to brush hair forward, leaning forward, and then toss your head and hair back to a standing position. If you wish, you can then smooth your hair into position where it will look much fuller than before.

Earthy Hair Variations

Parts

Becoming only to the very youthful face, a center part always spells Earthy. Side parts in conjunction with straight braids (especially the thin kind), pigtails, ponytails, or natural hair accessories can also work well. No part at all is Earthy when combined with the other elements of earthy hairstyling.

Curls

Natural waves and curls are wonderful; they can give that delightfully willful look. The smooth, shiny, fat kind of curl—typical of just off the hot rollers—does not give you the jungle look you're aiming for.

Permanents allowed to air dry, and other hairstyles that air dry to waves or frizz, look great in this image. Try braiding your wet hair, drying it, and wearing the crinkly lioness look without having to perm, it you are a little short on natural wave, curl, or body. Afros below chin length are very right for Earthy Face.

Bangs

Bangs should be brushed back from the face, toward the center back of the head. Wild and full is of course the best.

Upswept

Upswept hairstyles are seldom earthy in feeling, unless they reflect a hairstyle of a specific native ethnic group. Even then it will make your Earthy look either more glamorous or closer to classic in feeling. Hair pulled up at the crown of the head, with loose, skinny braids in a dangling ponytail, beaded at the ends, is an example of an earthy "upswept" styling.

Braids

Speaking of braids, they are Earthy when they are loose and skinny, long or short, straight not looped, mixed with loose hair, beaded, or corn-rowed.

Hair Colorings

Hair that appears sun-streaked, has reddish highlights, natural henna colors, or natural brown shades says Earthy and looks wonderful with that face.

Very metallic hair colors (for example, platinum blonde, salt and pepper, silver, or white) do not enhance this look. Hair that looks obviously dyed or altered can look a positive fright styled in the wild Earthy designs because of the difference in dyed-hair texture.

Hair that has been dyed dramatically to one solid, one-dimensional color is not Earthy. Sun-streaking, "Sun-In," luminizing, hennaing, and hair painting are all less thoroughly even. Thus they look more natural and casual—the ultimate in Earthy Image. If not overdone—and, importantly, suited to your coloring—these treatments can look fabulous!

Heavy frosting is overdone for this image, as it tends to look glamorous; but light frosting, if suited to your coloring, generally suits the earthy mood. Natural-substance highlighters or slight color enhancers—like henna with or without added spices; or lemon or chamomile rinses—are also good bets.

Hair Ornaments

Anything native and natural-looking goes. Instead of promoting control, your hair ornamentation may be used to bunch, gather, re-direct, or add volume to your hair (where you might have used, say, hot curlers for a different image) and to augment your garments for an even earthier aura.

Narrow, dangling hair ornaments are always earthy in design (unless antique European, such as Victorian). They are most attractive in natural objects and materials, and in earth-tone colors.

Ribbons and dress fabrics like velvet, lame and organdy used in your hair don't usually project that carefree feeling. Instead, try rope, shells, wooden beads, feathers, macrame, and braid for your hair ornaments. Try fabrics like corduroy, suede, and cotton. Vertical hanging designs are earthy in feeling.

Gypsy and "arty" bohemian scarves worn over your hair, or even a straw hat, if the weather is warm and you like the look, are fast, terrific answers to dyed locks or a hairstyle that can't seem to look "free" enough.

Headbands and Clips

Horizontal headbands, across the forehead, may be practical cloth ones—such as those worn for athletics, and by the American Indian—or decorative cloth or metal—such as those worn by Middle Eastern women or Wonder Woman.

Headbands, hairbands, barrettes, and ornamental combs will all work in Earthy hair, especially if they're made of natural or primitive materials or are designed to have something dangling from them—ribbons, tiny shells, or wooden beads, for example. However, if these accessories are used to control, they will project another image.

Materials can be leather and suede, fur, feathers, clay, terra cotta, "beaten metals," clay or glass beads, sandstone, wood, stones, cotton, gauze, muslin, terrycloth, and anything else along those lines that you can think of! Native hair ornaments, coordinated with matching jewelry, are particularly beautiful.

Accessorize Your Earthy Face

Earrings

- Natural luster of wood, "beaten" metals, or other like materials. No artificial, glittery, or dramatic colors, textures, or shapes.
- Narrow, dangling shapes create instant recognition. (Avoid them if they're European antique, Victorian or Edwardian, for instance.)
- Hoops in all varieties speak of Earthy, except the ½-inch diameter hoops that are wide and of plain, simple metal.
- The smallest pierced earrings—usually a ball, a bead, or a tiny stone in a metal setting—generally project earthiness, unless they are ¼-inch hearts or dainty garden flowers, which look Romantic.
- Best size: any, especially the smallest pierced earrings, the largest hoops, and medium-sized other shapes.

- Best materials: natural sources. Shell, wood, rope, straw, macrame, stone, feathers, clay or glass beads; "beaten" cooper, brass and silver; natural inlaid materials; animal hair or fur; and fabric.

Scarves

Try sailor knots, painter's ascots, and bandana-cornered neck scarves. Also Earthy: dangling and fringed shawls, and string ties. Top off your face with a gypsy-wrapped scarf if you like.

Necklines and Collars

Tasselled, fringed, crocheted, and gathered peasant necklines and collars are a fabulous earthy frame for your face and mood. Bateau, yoked, turtle-necked, and jewel necklines worn with natural jewelry, scarves, and collars can add to your Earthy aura. Unfinished necklines and collars may be Glamour, but more often are Earthy Image—more primitive in feeling.

Some Favorite Earthy Fabrics

Muslin, hemp, nubby wools and knits, suede, gabardines, poplin, denim, sailcloth, kettlecloth, Indian gauze, and "trunk" cotton or gauze are some of the perennial favorites.

Special Accessories for Earthy Image

- aviator sun—or clear—glasses, even if you don't need them! Or square, antique, wire-rimmed glasses for close-up work, even if you don't need them.
- thongs and native sandals
- large, straw hats and handbags
- fringed leather accessories
- rough-hewn leather belts, bags, and shoes
- headbands (across the forehead), sun visors
- anything with epaulettes on the shoulders, and safari or military cut

Earthy Magic by Candlelight

In the evening, you can wear pink with your Earthy Face. Generally a color to be avoided in Earthy, pink in the shade of "shrimp," a universal pink, adds radiance that earth tones lose as the sun goes down.

As with Classic and Romantic Images, you'll want a gentle hand when

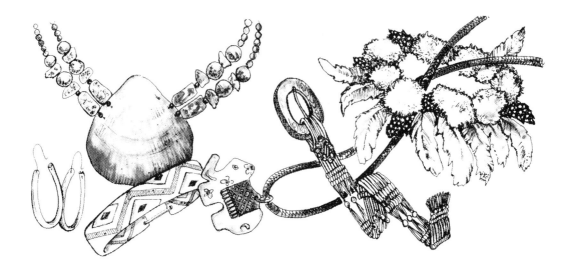

adjusting your Earthy Face to evening light. You don't want to lose the impact of your statement, and end up with a Glamour Face! Earthy is sultry enough to stand on its own in evening as well as daylight, and a Glamour Face would not coordinate with the Earthy evening fashions you've selected.

Turn up the volume of your Earthy Face statement for mystery! Try false eyelashes and stronger brow color for evening—the eyes and eyebrows will still be dominant, which is our Earthy key, so it's fine for sultry Earthy to mesmerize with strongly madeup eyes.

Dust your lids with a sheer film of charcoal powder. Charcoal adds depth that golds, bronzes, greens, cherrywoods, and ambers cannot achieve in evening light. Those warmly yellowish colors turn muddy rather than mysterious! You need your coolest earthy colors for evening light—cool shrimp and charcoal, for example. You also need the greater contrast the charcoal addition provides, because night light would otherwise flatten your features and drain away your vibrant color.

After applying your "sun-kissed" face color, add a hot shrimp pink creme color to evening "touch points": temples, cheekbones, collarbone indentions or cleavage, and earlobes.

Next dust your shoulders, collarbones and cheekbones with a lightly pearlized powder to add what appears to be the natural shimmer of moist, warm skin. This powder should be translucent so that it picks up your warm skin tones rather than obscuring your suntanned color, turning you pale.

Turn to the special section toward the end of this book for more on After-5:00 basics.

My Earthy Model Face

What Do I Need to Know Before I Begin?

When you apply more makeup than you'd want for your wholesome, down-to-earth Fast Face, your Earthy Face changes to become ever so slightly exaggerated. The look is less carefree and more exotic, erotic, and mysterious. The more exaggerated your makeup application, the stronger the impression of sensuality you will exude. Be sure to keep this in mind as you choose and apply cosmetics to your Earthy Face.

Foundation will need to create a dusky, creamy complexion. Darker skins can choose a color to match their natural tones, but if your skin is too pale, you'll need to choose colors that create a darker feeling.

Blend the outer edges well if your foundation shade is darker than your skin, so you don't appear to be wearing a masque. Choose warm tones with names like "dark, honey, warm, bronze, sunny, tan, or peachy." Don't use foundations, or bases referred to as "light, ivory, or rose."

Your skin should be healthy for this face, so use foundation sparingly, and choose another image if you're really blemished. Unhealthy or mature skin can look leathery in this image.

Highlighter isn't really necessary unless you'd like to use it along the jawbone to "square" the jaw. Use a shimmer-free product.

Concealers should be medium-to-dark colors and used more to cover blemishes than for any other purpose. Circles, veins, and spots are flaws; freckles, sunburn, beauty marks and moles are not blemishes in the Earthy Image.

Translucent Powder isn't necessary, and should be dark or medium in color if used. Apply sparingly, if at all. The same is true for **Powder Blushers.**

Eyebrow tools of all types are needed for your Earthy Imagery. You may want to use pencil and eyebrow powder along with your eyebrow brush. Whatever you choose, use a bold hand for an unruly look.

If your brows are too "civilized," try adding setting gel or hairspray to your eyebrow brush before you comb the brow. Then comb the eyebrow hairs, in the inner half of the brow, straight upward, letting the gel or spray dry in place.

You may need to make your brows look thicker, if you're wearing thin ones. A great way to add a stronger fullness to the brows is with dual products: eyebrow powder and pencil. The pencil is used to draw a straight line (even over the exposed skin) from end to end, and powder fills in the hair above it. Blend with your brush.

Brows cannot be too strong for this face. Close-set eyebrows that grow too close together produce an earthy effect. If you tweeze your brows to make them appear farther apart, you may want to fill in the natural growth area with brown color for this look.

The Earthy brow can be very prominent but trimmed slightly. Remove the hairs outside the natural brow line and below the frontal bone to open the eyes. Brush the inner half of the brows up and the outer half straight, horizontally out, across the face, toward the temple.

Eye makeup products of every variety can be employed for the sultry eyes of the Earthy Face. Pencils, kohl crayons, eyebrow powder, and eyeliners of every type serve to outline, elongate, and define the eye. Dusky powders and crayons enlarge and deepen eyes, increasing their smoky mystery.

The lower eyelids as well as the upper lids should be lined, to prevent a half-finished, unbalanced look. You can also line the inner lid between the lash and eyeball with a pencil for extra smolder.

Choose earth tones, dark colors, and smoky, hazy eye shadow and eyeliner shades. Iridescent (metallic shimmer) eye shadows can only be used if the colors are earth tones and you want sultry Earthy. Pastel, icy, and very cool metal colors work for other images—not for Earthy.

Blend all sharp makeup lines to achieve a subtly sultry look. Save the harsher lines for your Glamour look. As an example, compare the "mod" eye makeup of the young Audrey Hepburn (Glamour) against the "long, brown eye" of Sophia Loren (Earthy).

Don't curl mascaraed lashes; leave them spiked and straight. Mascara should be dark—either black or brown.

Remember to keep all eye makeup "lines" horizontal, not vertical. Think almond, slanted, cat-eyed.

Cheek Color. A gentle flush of color should be limited to the front of the face, not used on the side cheekbones. If your face doesn't have a "touched by the sun" color, smooth it on cosmetically. A blusher gel doesn't age the skin the way excess sun does, and it can look just as natural.

Liquid, gel, or creme rouge sticks are ideal, or mix your favorite creme color compact with a dab of moisturizer. Powder blushers can never produce the ideal Earthy glow. Just touch your cheeks (in the front of your face, vertically in line with your eyes), across the bridge of your nose, your temples, hairline, and maybe even your shoulders and collarbones. Cheek color never goes below the lobe of the ear.

Lips. Choose from an array of lip treatments. Add a clear or lightly earth toned gloss or lip balm. Or line your lips with a dusty pencil, blend the line, and add clear gloss.

In the 60's, a favored technique called for dusting full lips with powder, or barely covering them with foundation, then touching lightly with a moist-but-not-glossy earth color. This served to tone down the natural rosiness that colors the lips too strongly, detracting from the eyebrow-and-eye emphasis.

Whatever your choice, remember that lips do not dominate in this face. Lips may be full, but they are not darkly colored. Full lips have always been considered sensual, so they're especially appropriate for Earthy.

If you want carefree Earthy, instead, and have full lips that you want to make less noticeable, see how to correct too-full lips in the Contouring section. Or just remember to use light-color lipliner pencil and light lipstick on outer lip edges, and reduce gloss, which brings lips forward to the eye.

Earthy Model Face: Tool Checklist

Cosmetic Products

☐ Creme Flaw Concealer
  —medium-to-dark color
  —sheer, moist, lightweight
  —optional; don't use on freckles, beauty marks, etc.

☐ Foundation/Makeup Base
  —your darkest shade, up to 2 shades darker than your current natural skin tone
  —sheer, moist, lightweight

☐ Eyebrow Color
  —dry cake eyebrow powder, with stiff brush
  —pencil may also be used if desired
  —the darkest shade that still looks natural

☐ Mascara
  —brown, or brown-black

☐ Eyeliner
  —a medium-to-dark earth tone in your best colors
  —non-shimmer color for daytime Earthy
  —crayon, pencil or smudgeable liner product

☐ Eye Shadow
  —a medium and a dark earth tone (or your closest to earth tone colors)
  —matte (non-metalic) finish, unless you want sultry, evening Earthy
  —powders, crayons, creme sticks, etc.

☐ Face Color
  —liquid, gel, or creme cheek color
  —lightweight, moist, sheer to look like sun

☐ Lip Cosmetics
  —clear lip gloss, oil, or gel
  —or no color-to-light-color lip pomade (non-frost)
  —or ultra-sheer, barely earth-tone lipstick (moist, but non-frost)

☐ Lipliner Pencil
  —soft, earth tone, may be lip gloss color stick

Cosmetic Tools

☐ Makeup "silk" sponge
☐ Eyebrow brush
☐ "Vent" brush or perm pick for hair volume and fluff

Model Face—Earthy Formula

Eyebrow, Eyes, Sun-Kissed Complexion

1. Earthy Complexion

Lightly conceal actual blemishes with sheer, medium-to-dark concealer creme compact.

Lightly apply sheer, medium-to-dark foundation with makeup sponge.

Sheerly touch temples, forehead, chin, and nose with moist blusher for "sun-kissed" look. Slightly more heavily, touch cheek-to-cheek across the nose, but not carrying it out past the eyes to the hairline.

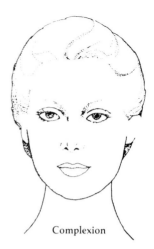

Complexion

2. Earthy Eyebrows

With eyebrow brush, brush the eyebrow hairs in the bulb of the eyebrow (the inner half of the eyebrow) straight upward.

Next, brush the outer half of the brow hairs straight across toward the temple/hairline. They should be as straight across and horizontal as the inner brows are straight up and vertical.

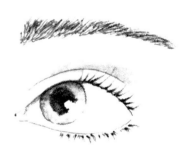

Straight Brow

Now fill in with eyebrow powder color if you need to straighten and embolden the brows.

If you have a typically arched eyebrow, start with the underside of the brow: color the skin with a straight line of color from the bulb to the outer half of the brow—filling in the arched bone with color to look like brow hair instead of bone.

If you need to, also square off the top edge, and the end of the inner half, of the brow with the same powder color. Then use your eyebrow brush to lightly brush the color on the skin to look like brow hairs, and to merge it with the underside edge of the actual brow.

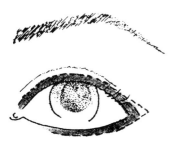

Eyeliner

3. Earthy Eyes

Line the upper and lower eyelids, wide and smoky and long. Wrap the color around the outer corner of the eye, where lower and upper eyelids meet. Carry the line straight out toward the temple just a bit to elongate if sultry is desired.

You may also line the inside lids, between lashes and eyeball, with dark pencil for extra smolder.

Dust either from upper lashes to the crease, between the top eyelid and the bone, or just in the crease itself, with your darkest eye shadow.

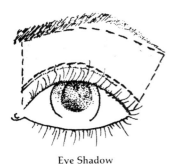

Eye Shadow

With medium, non-iridescent shadow, color the crease up to the eyebrow (or almost up to it if you want to leave a tiny bit of light underbrow-bone).

If you are going to apply either individual false eyelashes, or a string of them, now's the time. Remember to slant them up and out toward the temple for your sloe-eyed look.

Mascara your eye lashes, top and bottom.

If you want a particularly doe-eyed siren look, pay heavy attention to mascaraing your top lashes. Outer lashes are straight, not curled, and slant toward your temple. Less mascara is applied to your top inner lashes.

4. Earthy Wrap-Up

Add a final whisk of blusher gel or lip gloss if you feel you need it. Lean forward and then toss your head and hair back for some perky extra volume.

Now return to the Check-Out earlier in this Earthy Chapter for that final assurance that you've got the formula right and are projecting your best Earthy Image. Wasn't it easy to achieve?

Chapter 3

The Romantic Face

Setting the Mood

Your Romantic Image is the most subtly feminine of all your potential expressions of style. Its aura is soft, and gentle, and can be either youthful or womanly. When combined with dressing in styles reminiscent of another era, it radiates serenity.

Whether you're dressing in the current era or a past one, the components of this image should always appear "soft-focus." Feminine, graceful, gentle, ladylike, and dreamy are some of the ways in which you will be perceived in this image.

How Did Romantic Image Become So Popular?

Historically women have cherished jewelry, lace, and fabrics from preceding generations. Ultra-femininity has always been adored, but before the 20th Century, a romantic style was within the means of only the very wealthy. Ornate garments and adornments were costly; without the leisure and freedom afforded by affluence, women found it difficult to keep their skin soft, cared-for, and rosy by getting plenty of rest, fresh air, and exercise.

Modern women, however, have more time to pamper themselves a bit. They also have affordable fashions and fine skin care products. And instead of the enforced exposure to wind and weather experienced in earlier times, today's women can use fresh air and exercise to enhance their health and beauty.

Now pampered Romantic can be achieved by every woman!

The romantic look borrows from nature as well as from times past: lacy hearts, dreamy morning dew and colors, delicate ferns and dainty flowers are all models for romantic colors and design.

The joy of the Romantic Image is not only in what it says to others, but in the lift it gives by making you feel so ultra-feminine.

Famous Romantic Faces

Romantic faces have a fantasy quality because they're rarely pinned down to hard reality. Picture Gainsborough's lovely "Pinky," or the fairy tale Sleeping Beauty. In literature, we have the Bennett sisters in "Pride and Prejudice" (as well as Jane Austen herself!) and "Jane Eyre." A few modern examples are England's Queen Mother Elizabeth, Nastassia Kinski's film portrayal of "Tess of the D'Urbervilles.

Examples of famous women who have developed a romantic feeling for their particular image: Zsa Zsa Gabor, Arlene Dahl, Peggy Lee, Bernadette Peters, and, in a number of her films, Meryl Streep. Camera soft-focus is one way to attain the soft look of the Romantic Face. The makeup techniques in this book are another.

Why and When Do You Wear the Romantic Image?

You choose Romantic Image when you want to create a moment of soft spontaneity and romance. One romantic spirit is the aura of vulnerability. Another is kitten-like softness and a charming, ageless kind of innocence. You are so appealing, you disarm even the most cynical when you show your Romantic side.

When you and your skin are tired, and you want an easy, fresh style, Romantic can help you look and feel younger. Romantic is kinder to you than the other images. It's not a lot of makeup, so it's also appropriate for evening makeovers where you'll be at home but don't want full "war paint." Romantic is always there for you when you need a quick makeover for your off-work hours, when Earthy isn't your mood at the moment.

What about those hot, humid days when you pull your hair up or back, even if it's not your regular hairstyle? Long or medium hair is a natural for that impromptu Romantic look.

On the practical side, if you are heavier than your usual weight, Romantic image suits your rounded face and figure, making you appear luscious and "waiting to be picked."

You may not be a sun-tanning enthusiast. Perhaps you have nice, soft, or pale skin and would like to keep it that way? Romantic is the nice and easy face to slip on your pale complexion for casual or dressy times.

You may have naturally mild, gentle coloring and features. Many women with such coloring know that they are, what are now called in popular terminology, *"Spring/Light-Bright/Sunlights* and *Summer/Gentle/Sunlights"* You will find to your delight that Romantic plays up your features making the most of their gentleness rather than covering it with strong makeup that overshadows your fairy-tale fairness. A little makeup goes a long way on you. This delicate Romantic Face will surely become one of your all-time favorites!

Another woman who will especially appreciate Romantic Image: the soft-skinned mature face is made to look younger in both spirit and texture with Romantic Face

Romantic is as flattering to young women as it is to mature ones, to innocent personalities or moods, and to the rounder face and figure. It also flatters any age.

And by the way, men absolutely adore this image. Try it on someone who interests you; he may ask you to marry him on the spot! If you've long since found your loved one, try it and see if you don't recreate some precious memories.

There will always be a time in every woman's life when she desires this image—if not for a man, than surely for her own joy of expression.

Romantic Image: for the soft and feminine you.

Where Do You Wear the Romantic Image?

This image is especially suited to your romantic moments—special interludes and times, including evenings. Warm feelings at parties, picnics, dating, intimate dinners for two, anniversaries, close-family gatherings, holidays, church services, and vacations all take on an added glow with your Romantic Image. Try announcing an expected bundle of joy in this look for that misty moment, feeling cuddled, protected, and cherished by your loved ones.

Obviously a gentleman is part of the picture in a lot of these settings; but not always. *Maternal* feelings and familial enjoyment also suit the mood of Romantic Image.

Romantic is the ultimate image to wear to weddings whether you are the bride, a member of the procession, or a guest. In fact, Romantic is so beautiful for the marriage occasion, a special section in this Romantic chapter has been devoted to the Romantic Bride and her all-important day.

Go charmingly Romantic, also, to events like engagement, wedding, and baby showers. Pregnant women have such a bloom about them that this dewy, hopeful image is better suited to that precious time of your life than the other images.

For one of those old sepia-colored photographs, or a costume for a masquerade party, or theatricals, you'll need a face to match the patina of the garments. Romantic is so right; you've seen it in every scrapbook.

On a more serious note, if you want to stay low-key and low-profile in a group situation, wear the Romantic image. People will want to protect you and will not try to advance you to leadership, extra involvement, or high-profile activities.

Romantic is demure and ladylike. The first time you meet relatives you don't know, including your fiance's parents, they would probably be thrilled to have the Romantic you as their first impression. Romantic Image pleases almost everyone!

What are the Characteristics of the Romantic Face?

Bring to mind the essence of this image by envisioning the pastoral maidens or princesses of your childhood storybooks. In cultures everywhere, this maid symbolizes romance. The French Impressionists loved to paint her.

The Romantic Face lacks artifice even if you're up to your neck in ruffles or you're covered in row upon row of lace. Unlike the other images, no particular feature of the face is emphasized to dominate! This is a total departure from the other formulas.

The look is fresh and wide-eyed. Complexions are soft and clear. Even your hair is fluffy and soft-focus. If you can manage to look rosy and moist as if you have just awakened from a refreshing nap, you'll have it. Think in terms of:

- creamy, milky, soft, dewy skin
- all features in soft focus; not one dominating over the others, and no appearance of harsh or strong features here
- rosy, pink cheeks and lips
- round, wide-eyed, doe-eyed

Modern stressful lifestyles have brought a resurgence in interest in a softened kind of feminine beauty for special occasions or daily wear. Such a look implies that she "stops and smells the roses," a happy prospect to others who don't.

Introducing You to the Romantic Image Formula

Do I Have Time for It?

Romantic Face makeup is second only to the most carefree image, Earthy, in its ease of application. It's fast, easily applied, and because all the makeup "edges" are blurred, it doesn't require great skill, time, or complicated tools.

You don't use any makeup techniques that promote angular bones, like Classic, or sharply defined color, shape, or texture, like Glamour. Nothing dramatic is applied, so you have no "edges" to even out.

Although the number of makeup items to be used is small, without the right cosmetics and tools you cannot achieve this face.

For speed, when your hair is long, shoulder- or medium-length, this may be your first choice of image. You merely pile up your hair in a knot on the top of your head, styling your hair as quickly as you style your Romantic Face.

Women with short, straight hair will spend a little more time, because they'll probably need curls. Plan them in advance—set them at night or while you fix breakfast—you can pull your look together nearly as quickly as those with longer hair.

Lastly, when you're embarking on an evening out, and you have 30 minutes to spend instead of the usual 5 or 10, design your hair to become a really beautiful frame for your face. Artfully arranging tendrils, waves, braids, curls, knots and ribbons can become as complex as you like, and as rewarding.

Since your makeup is fast and simple, any time you lavish will be on your hair, or a soak in a fragrant bubble bath to build the mood, or perhaps even buttoning hundreds of tiny buttons!

Does Romantic Image Work on Me?

Well-chosen colors, garments, and hair arrangements are the essential elements in creating this image. Although the pale hair and skin tones typically associated with romantic styles are easiest to work with, even those with gypsy-dark features can wear Romantic Face. They just need to follow the Romantic Face formula, and choose colors, garments, and hairstyles appropriate to the Romantic Image.

In comparison to the other faces, your Romantic Face is the most easily "lost" when not well framed by carefully selected garments and hairstyles.

Facial shape is not particularly important, although round, heart-shaped, and oval are easiest. Round faces, contrary to popular belief, are beautiful in this rounded, peaches-and-cream style. Not only does it look lovely, but this facial shape makes cosmetic application even faster and more effective. The only caution here is that the round faces that accompany rounded figures can look fussy in an ornate hairstyle. Choose a soft-focus style instead of overabundant or small, sausage curls.

The Romantic Image is particularly lovely and fast to produce when face and figure are either very youthful or not thin to the point of gaunt.

If you are thin and ascetic looking, you can achieve Romantic by wisely emphasizing your fragile quality. Flowing gowns will flatter your slenderness, and flowers in the hair of a frail wood nymph can be charming with her Romantic Face peeping out from beneath.

Coloring and skin tones can assist you in achieving this image. Romantic best suits the natural "bunny" with pale eyes, eyelashes, and brows. Naturally rosy cheeks are also a plus, even the overbright flush caused by some medications.

Pale or rosy-cheeked *"Autumn/Muted/Sunset"*; *"Spring/Light-Bright/Sunlight"*; or *"Summer/Gentle/Sunlight"* coloring will need very little cosmetic assistance. Since the end product is most importantly soft, your light or smoky pastels and hazy tints in cosmetics and clothing are a must.

Although these creamy skin types with light-to-medium eyebrow colors find this beauty formula easiest, every woman can enjoy her own variation of Romantic Face. Heavy, dark eyebrows make a glaring slash of strong color and sharp angle on an otherwise softened face. They need to be tidied and powdered to lighten.

By enhancing her natural coloring with drama, the golden, brown or dark-skinned romantic will achieve all the romance of her pale counterpart. Instead of rosy-cheeked auras, theirs will be one of golden or ebony beauty. Makeup application and hairstyling will not differ. They will still keep all features equal in dominance so that none appears strong. Features will be as soft in feeling as can be achieved. Only the choice of clothing and colors will differ.

Skin type is less important than its texture and health. Very blemished skin is better in the Faces that offer greater coverage. Perhaps the skin care covered in the special section of this book will help bring the skin back into good condition, making Romantic suitable in the future. Pore-less seeming skin is perfect for Romantic (although makeup can work miracles in that direction!)

Fair freckles should be gently covered, although very fair, freckled looks are wonderful in Romantic with just a hint of blurring of them. They look especially charming in this face if you are youthful and fair. Sunburned or very tanned skin needs to wait for another day.

Romantic Face spans all age groups more gracefully than any other image. It enhances the teenager without overshadowing her never-to-be-seen-again budding bloom. She looks her prettiest and is still natural for her age. This quality recaptures something of that young beauty for every age beyond young womanhood, yet never looks inappropriately youthful on the mature woman. This is because it is so subtle that it always appears as the wearer's own natural bloom.

To summarize the basics for creating your Romantic Face:
- Complexion—creamy, flushed with health, dew-drenched
- Eyebrows—subdued, rounded
- Cheekbones—"apple cheeks"; rounded
- Lips—rosebud
- Colors: soft, pastel, hazy, opaque. Especially pinks, lavender, soft greens, ivory
- Hair—rounded styles, uncontrolled but not tomboyish-looking or unkempt, old-fashioned overtones
- Soft-focus

Romantic Fast Face

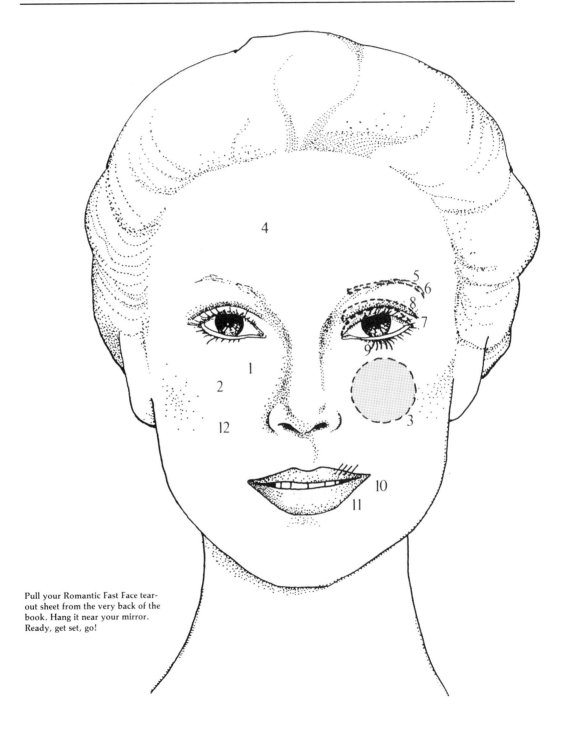

Pull your Romantic Fast Face tear-out sheet from the very back of the book. Hang it near your mirror. Ready, get set, go!

Although Romantic Face appears unmade up, remember that it does require makeup; it's not just two circles of rouge or a slash of lipstick on a pale face. Instead of falling back on old makeup habits, try Romantic a few times; you'll find that suddenly it will feel as easy as your former makeup technique.

Ready to Try on Your Romantic Face?

Whether you use the Fast Face or the Model Face makeover, the more closely you follow this Romantic-appeal formula, the more Romantic the spell you cast will be—from the first moment.

—Fast Face—Romantic Formula

All Features Equal

Complexion

1 Quickly cover flaws and dark circles with light concealer stick
2 Blend your palest sheer foundation lightly with sponge
3 Rouge the cheek "apples"; blend well into small area with sponge
4 Dust face with translucent powder (only lightly on cheek "apples")

Eyebrows

5 Brush into rounded shape with eyebrow brush; avoid coloring them
6 Smooth your translucent powder onto rounded brows (unless already extremely light)

Eyes

7 Draw wide, domed eyeliner with sheer, neutral crayon; smudge to blur its edges
8 Add sheer, pastel color to the crease; smudge to blur
9 No mascara, or barely touch light-colored mascara to top and bottom center lashes only (starry eyes)

Lips

10 Cover lightly with foundation
11 Add opaque, sheer, light color in rose or peach

Finishing Touch

12 Pat face with sea sponge wetted then squeezed "dry" (to add dewy moisture and to "set" makeup to last)

The Total Look

Pulling It All Together in the Romantic Image

1. Creamy, milky, peaches-and-cream, and roses-in-your-cheeks complexion. Flaws covered but appearance of little makeup. Dewy, pore-less seeming skin.
2. No features dominate; the entire face is in soft focus.
3. All features look rounded, rosy: apple cheeks, doe-like eyes, full, softened lips, rounded, unobtrusive brows, and fine lashes.
4. Romantic is characterized by light to medium, gentle colors—especially pastels. They can be either hazy and smoky, or clear with a non-metallic yet dewy finish. Dreamy, not dark.

Eyebrows
1. Light, or powdered; rounded
2. Not strong; downplayed
3. Rounded highlighting

Cheeks
1. Not bony; rounded
2. Young, round apple-cheek flush

Lips
1. Rosy, peachy
2. Light-to-medium, opaque colors
3. Dewy, but low shine
4. Bow or rosebud style

Complexion
1. Milky, creamy, fair
2. Flawless and pore-less looking
3. Moist and dewy, but not shiny

Hair
1. Old-fashioned styles, such as topknots, "Gibson Girl," or braids. Any length.
2. Rounded styles, with escaping wisps, fuzzies, tendrils, curls (graceful or fussy)
3. No sculpted, angular lines
4. Accents: tiny, feminine, light, and airy

Eye Makeup
1. Minimal, gentle
2. Pastels, clear or smoky (especially aqua, purples, pinks and peaches)
3. Domed, rounded eyelid, barely darkened

Ornaments
1. Tiny, diminutive jewelry, ½ inch diameter or less, unless antique)
2. Not angular or dramatic
3. Antique, ribbons, lace, floral
4. Pearly, beaded, brushed gold, filigree silver, etc.

Garments
1. Old world influence
2. Soft, flowing pastel colors
3. Fabrics: light, soft, often sheer, lacy, gauzy, or angora
4. Dainty, pristine, delicate
5. Small-pattern prints, especially floral

Buzz Words
1. Peaches-n-cream skin, doe eyes
2. Apple cheeks, rosebud lips
3. Old-fashioned styles
4. Soft, light natural fabrics
5. Dreamy, light colors
6. Soft-focus, airy, lady-like
7. Gentle, rounded, non-madeup
8. Nails: light, rounded, not long
9. Fragrance: light, feminine, maybe sweet, fruity, floral, potpourri

Check It Out, And Go!

Is your "balance of power" correct for Romantic Image—all features equally emphasized? Is it all soft-focused, and with no obvious makeup?

Lipstick not too dark? Not too white? Lips soft and moist, but not shiny/glossy?

Brows rounded, and not making any strong statement? Eyes rounded, and makeup gentle?

Apple cheeks? Rouge still there? (sometimes absorbs quickly)

Complexion looks flawless and your palest? No dry or caking areas?

You look enchanting.

The Romantic Color Palette

To create a romantic look, your best color choices are soft and dreamy, gentle and dewy, and best in light-to-medium intensity color range.

Difficult to use in projecting a romantic look are: bright, brilliant, shiny, shimmery, or dry and flat colors, which all tend to make an Earthy or Glamour statement.

Your "coolest" colors are best. If you know that you are a *Spring/Light-Bright/Sunlight*, keep in mind that your "coolest" soft pastels and least vivid colors are perfect. If you know that you are a *Winter/Contrast/Sunrise*, your light, icy shades with a pink or rose undertone are good, but be careful that icy color isn't in a wet or shiny fabric. If you know that you are an *Autumn/Muted/Sunset*, your delicate shades, such as fawn and celery, are most romantic. *Summer/Gentle/Sunlight*, with the most romantic colors in its key, is a seemingly endless rainbow of suitable colors from which to choose!

Any type of natural coloring can create a Romantic mood. Simply choose your flattering colors and:

Think soft, cool, dreamy, misty, swirling

Some Suggested Colors

Black	Warm, clear beige
Icy violet	Light, warm violet
Icy lemon	Buttercream
Icy lime	Light, warm aqua
Icy blue	Medium, warm turquoise
Seafoam (lightest) green	Light, clear peach
Pink icing	Warm, seashell pink
Lavender frost	Blushing peach
Crystal grey	Ivory
Pearl grey	Cream
Lavender	Jade green
Robin's egg blue	Celery
Robin's egg green	Sepia
Rosy beige	Oyster
Pink, light cocoa	Doe-skin
Mauve	Copper
Powder pink	Puce
Powder blue	Champagne
Pink rose	Ash rose
Off-white	Ecru

Romantic Sample Makeup Color Schemes

Icy Pink Scheme

Concealer: "Vert," cool blue-green (white) base

Foundation: Cool—ivory, bisque, "rose"

Face Powder: Light, translucent, no frost

Creme Rouge: Rose, pink, bright pink

Lipstick: Non-metallic—pastel pink, bright (sheer) burgundy

Mascara: none or sable, no "midnight" dark colors

Eye Shadow: Non-metallic—icy violet, icy aqua, icy green, powder blushes in the creme rouge colors, above, used as eye shadow only

Warm Carnation Scheme

Concealer: Light, warm, creamy

Foundation: Light, warm, ivory or bisque, two shades lighter than skin

Face Powder: light, translucent, no frost

Creme Rouge: Clear, hot carnation, warm, pastel pink, soft clear coral pink

Lipstick: Clear, hot carnation, warm pastel pink, coral pink

Mascara: none, or clear honey brown

Eye Shadow: Warm medium violet, pastel yellow-green (not icy), soft, warm periwinkle, pastel turquoise; powder blushers in the creme rouge colors, above, used as eye shadow only

For the information of the serious color student:

Clear, Cold, Blue-based
Winter/Contrast/Sunrise

Clear, Warm, Yellow-based
Spring/Light-Bright/Sunlight

Sample Makeup Color Schemes

Powder Pink Scheme

Concealer: Soft, creamy white or lightest becoming shade

Foundation: Cool—rose, ivory bisque, or cane—2 shades lighter than skin

Face Powder: Light, translucent, no frost

Creme Rouge: Powder, rosy, or pastel pink, or dusty burgundy

Lipstick: Pastel, carnation with blue cast, or sheer dusty plum

Mascara: Violet, lavender, or rose brown

Eye Shadow: Aqua, rosy brown, heather purples and lavender

Apricot Scheme

Concealer: Warm, oyster white, or lightest yellow-based shade

Foundation: Warm, yellow-based—beige, oyster, cane, or ivory—2 shades lighter than skin

Face Powder: Light, translucent, no frost

Creme Rouge: Apricot; or deep peach

Lipstick: Apricot, peach or cool, sheer coffee

Mascara: Light brown

Eye Shadow: Jade, turquoise, (smoky), periwinkle blue, light pumpkin

For the information of the serious color student:

Cloudy, Cool, Blue-based
Summer/Gentle/Sunlight

Cloudy, Warm, Yellow-based
Autumn/Muted/Sunset

Romantic Hair

De-emphasize modern angles, precision-cut lines, or blunt cuts with curls, fluff, and ornaments to create that old-world innocence.

With this restriction, hair can then be any length and worn either up or down. Hair that curls is the essence of Romantic. This allows women of all ages to achieve romantic hairstyling, since there are many styles of curls from those for the very youngest who tend to prefer long and curly, to the most mature, who tend to prefer short hair with medium-sized permed curls.

Additionally, any combination of curly, wispy bangs; hair knots and a few loose tendrils; French or medium-to-thick, rounded braids; and softly fuzzy curls usually suits the Romantic Image. And if you are really in the mood, adding Renaissance ribbons and/or tiny Victorian baby's breath and flowers, a string of seed pearls, or an abundance of softly escaping tendrils and "fuzz" in theme with your garments will be appealingly romantic.

Long, flowing, crimped locks are best worn with light, flowing garments of Greek, Roman, Middle Eastern, or medieval influence. The Gibson-Girl topknot perched on rounded full hair suits Victorian high-necked, lacy clothing.

Short hair can be pin-curled, or curled with a curling iron or rollers, to free it from its precision-cut look and to restyle it for a softer, romantic look.

Textures

Romantic hair is enchantingly feminine—with loose cascading, fuzzy or round curls, waving swirls, or escaping ringlets and tendrils. Romantic hair is never tight or perfectly tidy.

Lengths

Any length, except extremely short "little boy" and cropped cuts, can be converted to a romantic style. Even with the shortest hair, however, curls, tiny ribbons, flowers, and accessories can be used to simulate the romantic aura—for example, a narrow ribbon tied around your head with a bows at the top is charming when worn with your at-home lingerie.

General Designs

Haircut designs that are obviously dramatic, asymmetric, or extremely short reduce the clarity of the image you are trying to produce. It is the modern line that undermines the feeling rather than the hair length itself.

Hairstyles should be feminine, soft, and as "fuzzy" in silhouette as is becoming to you. Keep your accessorizing non-dramatic in line, texture, and color; fussy is fine, but if done on too big a scale can look dramatic.

Here is a simple chart of some romantic hairstyle variations you may wish to experiment with.

Romantic Hair Variations

Parts

Center parts are Romantic. A word of caution: they're unflattering after about age 8, unless you have perfectly symmetrical features, a receding chin, or a round face. Single, side parts are more Classic or Glamour in feeling. If you like a slightly classical kind of romantic style, keep them in mind.

Double side parts (one on each side of the head), frequently used with braiding, are very romantic.

Curls

All curls have the potential to appear Romantic. Exceptions are: dramatic short guiches close to the ear (Glamour), and highly-controlled, medium curls swept off the face and evenly surrounding the head (Classic).

Tight curls should be combed out to be looser and less controlled, or they should be fuzzed. Body waves are best when set to become slightly tighter—large curls. They can be gathered anywhere on the head or used to frame the face.

Cascading, dangling, swirling, curly, fuzzy, or escaping locks are deliciously feminine. Whatever style curl you wear, keep them loose and soft-focus.

Afro-style tight perms with a sleek, round silhouette are Classic or Glamour rather than Romantic.

Bangs

Bangs can be an important Romantic statement. It's easy to convert any style bang to Romantic Image, whether spare or thick. Simply set them with curlers into wispy tendrils or full, face-framing curls.

Braids

Rounded braids can be beautifully romantic. Try French braiding, or braided knots of hair. Braids that frame the face (or cling to the head with a rounded, non-angular silhouette) are lovely.

Knots

Knots of hair, either smooth rolls or fat braids, are best placed on top of the head or at the back crown of the head. (Nape knots look classic and side knots glamour, so avoid them.) Knots look even more romantic with escaping wisps and tendril curls.

Upswept

Upswept styles can always be converted for a romantic feeling. Reduce back-combing and teasing, and use soft, loose, non-sleek lines with plenty of escaping locks for your most romantically upswept look. Add braids or accessories for very special times.

Hair Colorings

It is difficult to create a "soft-focus" feeling with dramatic, obviously dyed hair. Natural hair color is best, and if you can add strawberry or red overtones subtly (even temporarily), you'll add more warmth to your Romantic Image.

Natural flaxen or blonde hair, or light or dark hair with red and strawberry overtones, are the most romantic hair colorings. However, if those overtones don't suit your coloring, they're not worth adding, because they'll tamper with your natural beauty that is, after all, the essence of the Romantic Look.

If you'd like to try a temporary hint of one-night brush-in color powder, color spray, or color-rinse for a special occasion, keep to rose tones if you're blue-based (*"Winter/Contrast/Sunrise"*, or *"Summer/Gentle/Sunlight"*). Keep to warm, honey tones if you're yellow-based (*"Spring/Light-Bright/Sunlight"*, or *"Autumn/Muted/Sunset"*).

Hair Ornaments

Tiny ornaments, like seed pearls, jet beads, baby's breath, dried flowers, rosebuds, tatting, special lace trims, braids, and very narrow ribbons can be wound through the hair or used to frame the face to great advantage. They evoke a feeling of exquisite beauty and are usually not worn with very contemporary garments.

One caution about tiny hair ornaments or jewelry: if you have a large head or very angular bone structure, the tiniest of these extra additions should be avoided, as they throw you into noticeably sharp contrast.

Other natural, old-fashioned, and traditional materials—like cotton, velvet, tortoise shell, ivory, gold or silver trims, faux pearls, and horn—are best. However, shells, feathers, stone and other natural materials are Earthy Image, so be alert not to cross over into these.

Hair Combs

A must for a truly Victorian look, hair combs can be used with contemporary clothes, too, for a useful as well as decorative romantic touch. They should be made of natural materials, for Romantic, like the ones described above. They can shape the hair, or capture it to leave many free hair ends, contributing to a whimsical look.

Accessorize Your Romantic Face

Earrings

- No dramatic or vivid colors or shapes
- Nothing larger than 1 inch, unless it's antique (or faux antique)—the smaller the better
- Nothing dangling unless it's antique (or antique-look)
- Best size: less than ½-inch across
- Best shapes: any non-modern; rounded edges best (hoops are never Romantic Image). Designs of hearts or garden flowers are Romantic.
- Best materials: china, pearl, ivory semi-precious stones, tortoise, gold (especially brushed), silver (especially filigree), inlay, and jet
- Pierced earrings ¼-inch or less in Romantic shapes.

Scarves

Soft-flowing, sheer fabrics, that drape gently, can be eminently Romantic. Ruffled, fluted, pleated, and fanned scarves can look romantic. A light-weight, old-world, lacy-crochet, or organza ruffle type of shawl can complete an old-fashioned ensemble.

Instead of a scarf, add a ribbon—with or without cameo brooch or dangling locket—at your neck. Water-marked taffeta or grosgrain, or velvet, are especially nice for this touch.

Your New Image in 8 Minutes or Less!

8 Minute Makeovers is a beauty book *and* an image book. Why look just OK when, in 8 minutes or less, you can look more beautiful and more interesting. In no time you can project a style to match your mood, your goals, or your setting.

Choose Classic to look refined and understated; choose Earthy to look sensuous and carefree; choose Romantic to look soft and feminine; and choose Glamour to look dramatic and chic.

These color pages will show you, step-by-step, how to achieve these four beautiful Images. So turn the page and step into a new Look!

Clare Miller

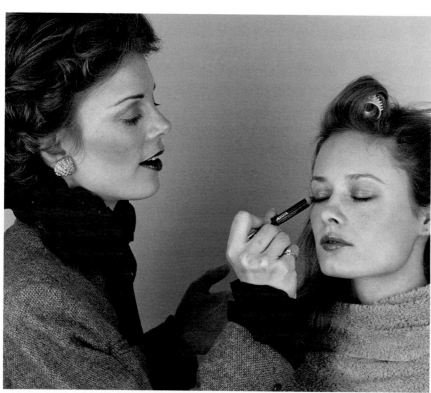

Photographs courtesy AZIZA COSMETICS by Prince Matchabelli

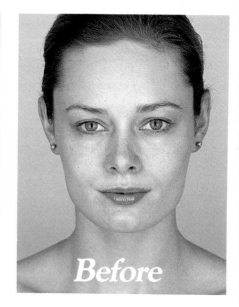

Before

Here's the model with no makeup at all.

And at left, I am using makeup to transform her from plain to gorgeous.

Turn the page to see how fabulous she looks in each of the four Images.

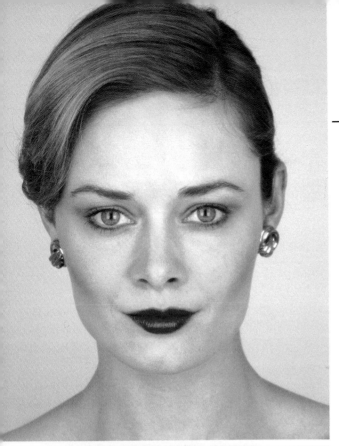

The Classic Face

Your Classic Face projects elegance and refinement, power and assurance, quality and integrity, understatement and timelessness. Classic is conservative, tailored, and clean. Toned down for town-and-country sports or toned up for business, your Classic Face is appropriate no matter where you go.

You'll want to wear Classic for interviews, business travel, graduations, civic meetings, resorts, and as a participant or spectator of sports activities.

The key to Classic is the balance of eyebrow, cheekbone, and lip emphasis.

See Plates D & E.

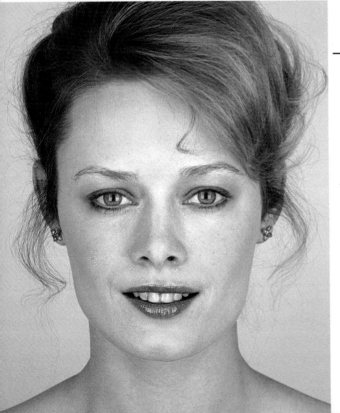

The Romantic Face

Your Romantic Face is subtly feminine. Romantic is soft and gentle, serene and graceful, demure and delicate, fresh and wide-eyed. Romantic projects vulnerability, innocence, and romance. It can help you look and feel younger.

You'll want to wear Romantic for intimate dinners for two, parties, dates, and when meeting your lover's parents. Romantic is the perfect face for brides and wedding guests, too.

The key to Romantic is soft focus — no one feature dominates this face.

See Plates F & G

If you'd like to see what cosmetics were used to achieve each Image, turn to the Cosmetics List at the back of the book.

The Earthy Face

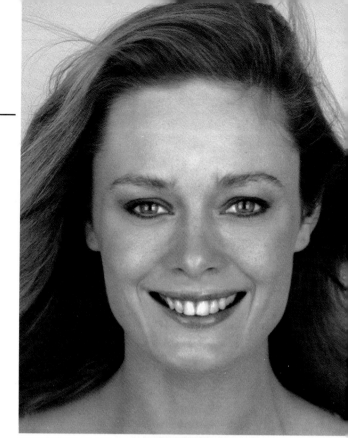

Your Earthy Face is casual and sensual, wild and sultry, healthy and sun-tanned, relaxed and sporty. Earthy projects your fun-loving and adventurous side. Unruly and capricious work in Earthy.

You'll want to wear Earthy for informal gatherings, beach vacations, running, camping, and to look arty. And wear Earthy if you want men to see your blatant temptress appeal!

The key to Earthy is eye and eyebrow emphasis.

See Plates H & I

The Glamour Face

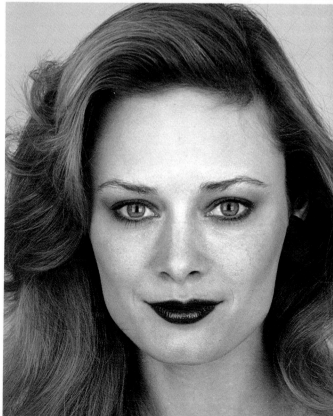

Your Glamour Face is pizazz. Glamour is sexy, sophisticated, dramatic, trendy, daring, and dazzling. Glamour can be severe and high fashion. Glamour is the most popular Image for evening. It's also the best Image to complement strikingly colored hair and very high fashion clothing and hairstyles.

You'll want to wear your Glamour Face anytime you want to make a splash — entertaining, at parties, discos, jazz clubs, the opera. You may want the Glamour Look if you work in the fashion/beauty industry, advertising, modeling, acting, music, or dance.

The key to Glamour is eye and lip emphasis.

See Plates J & K

Photographs courtesy AZIZA COSMETICS by Prince Matchabelli

PLATE C

The Classic Palette

Your best Classic colors are true, traditional, of medium intensity, and not exaggerated light or dark. Think medium, true, opaque, and traditional.

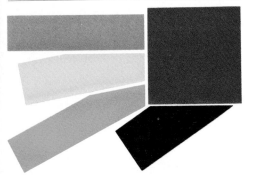

Autumn
Muted
Sunset

If your color key is Autumn, Muted, or Sunset, here are some of your Classic colors:
• Windsor teal
• camel
• old gold
• bright hunter
• scarlet rust

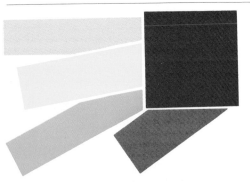

Spring
Light-Bright
Sunlight

If your color key is Spring, Light-Bright, or Sunlight, some of your Classic colors are:
• light clear navy
• buff
• banana
• medium spring green
• coral bright

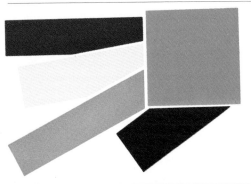

Summer
Gentle
Sunlight

If your color key is Summer, Gentle, or Sunlight, some of your Classic colors are:
• Wedgwood blue
• greyed navy
• light lemon yellow
• deep blue green
• cordovan

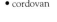

Winter
Contrast
Sunrise

If your color key is Winter, Contrast, or Sunrise, some of your Classic colors are:
• true blue
• light flannel grey
• primary yellow
• emerald
• ruby red

The Classic Image

Classic is elegant, refined, understated, timeless, conservative, and always appropriate.

Remember to balance the Classic Face with a hairstyle that's neat, shiny, healthy, and symmetrical. Hair should be shoulder-skimming or shorter.

Classic jewelry and accessories are tailored, medium to small in size, and not too dramatic.

Classic clothing is conservative, tailored, and neat.

Step-by-Step

The Goal: complexion, eyebrow, cheekbone, and lip emphasis

Complexion
1. Perfect it: cover circles, blemishes (and lighten eyelid centers) with light concealer stick

Eyebrows
2. Shape into Classic Arch with cake eyebrow powder
3. Brush brow and run the eyebrow brush along top of brow to return any wild hairs back to brow
4. Highlight underneath brow, its full length

Cheekbones
5. Dust face with a pad of translucent powder (loose or pressed compact)
6. Brush powder blusher into cheek hollow, blend with sponge

Lips
7. Add opaque, medium lip color — inside or up to lip line

Option Touches
8. A light coat of mascara
9. Medium eye color in crease of eye (just above lid)
10. Lipliner pencil inside lip line (before lip color)
11. Extra whisk with face powder pad

Illustrations by Christine Turner

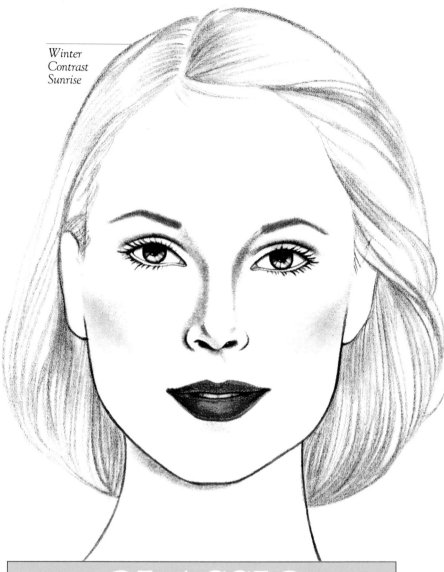

Winter Contrast Sunrise

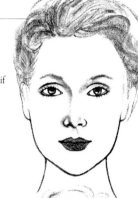

Autumn Muted Sunset
Here's the Classic Look if you're an Autumn, Muted, or Sunset.

Spring Light-Bright Sunlight
Here's the Classic Look if you're a Spring, Light-Bright, or Sunlight.

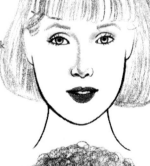

Summer Gentle Sunlight
Here's the Classic Look if you're a Summer, Gentle, or Sunlight.

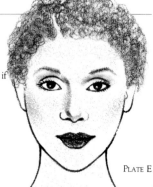

Winter Contrast Sunrise
Here's the Classic Look if you're a Winter, Contrast, or Sunrise.

CLASSIC

The Formula

1. The Classic triangle: eyebrows, cheekbones, and lips
2. Flawless-seeming, pale complexion
3. Opaque, medium intensity colors
4. Understated, symmetrical, and traditional hairstyle and accessories

PLATE E

The Romantic Palette

Your best Romantic colors are soft, pastel and misty. They're best in light to medium intensity.

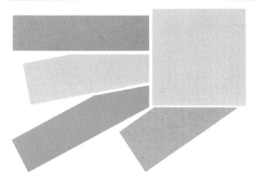

Autumn
Muted
Sunset

If your color key is Autumn, Muted, or Sunset, here are some of your Romantic colors:

• soft jade
• lilac haze
• doe-soft beige
• dusty jade
• dusty rose

Spring
Bright-Light
Sunlight

If your color key is Spring, Bright-Light, or Sunlight, here are some of your Romantic colors:

• warm sweet turquoise
• blushing peach
• orange sherbet
• bright new grass
• warm seashell peach

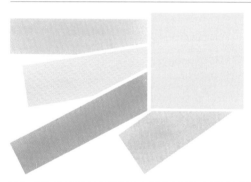

Summer
Gentle
Sunlight

If your color key is Summer, Gentle, or Sunlight, here are some of your Romantic colors:

• dusty pastel blue
• misty lavender
• robin's egg green
• crocus bud
• pastel rose

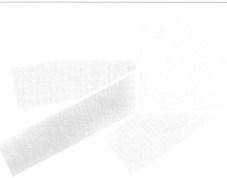

Winter
Contrast
Sunrise

If your color key is Winter, Contrast, or Sunrise, here are some of your Romantic colors:

• iced aqua
• iced lemon
• icy pink
• iced violet
• iced limeade

The Romantic Image

Romantic is soft, feminine, innocent, and delicate.

Romantic hair is curled or waved and creates a rounded style. Its length can be short, medium, or long.

Romantic jewelry and accessories are small, pearly, beaded, antique, filigree, ribbons, and lace.

Romantic clothing is soft and flowing, often sheer, often printed, delicate, floral, and dainty.

Step-by-Step

The Goal: all features equal

Complexion

1. Quickly cover flaws and dark circles with light concealer stick
2. Blend your palest sheer foundation lightly with sponge
3. Rouge the cheek "apples"; blend well into small area with sponge
4. Dust face with translucent powder (only lightly on cheek "apples")

Eyebrows

5. Brush into rounded shape with eyebrow brush; avoid coloring them
6. Smooth your translucent powder onto rounded brows (unless already extremely light)

Eyes

7. Draw wide, domed eyeliner with sheer, neutral crayon; smudge to blur edges
8. Add sheer, pastel color to crease, smudge to blur
9. No mascara, or barely touch light-colored mascara to top and bottom center lashes only (starry eyes)

Lips

10. Cover lightly with foundation
11. Add opaque, sheer, light color in rose or peach

Finishing Touch

12. Pat face with sea sponge wetted then squeezed dry (to add dewy moisture and to set makeup to last)

Illustrations by Christine Turner

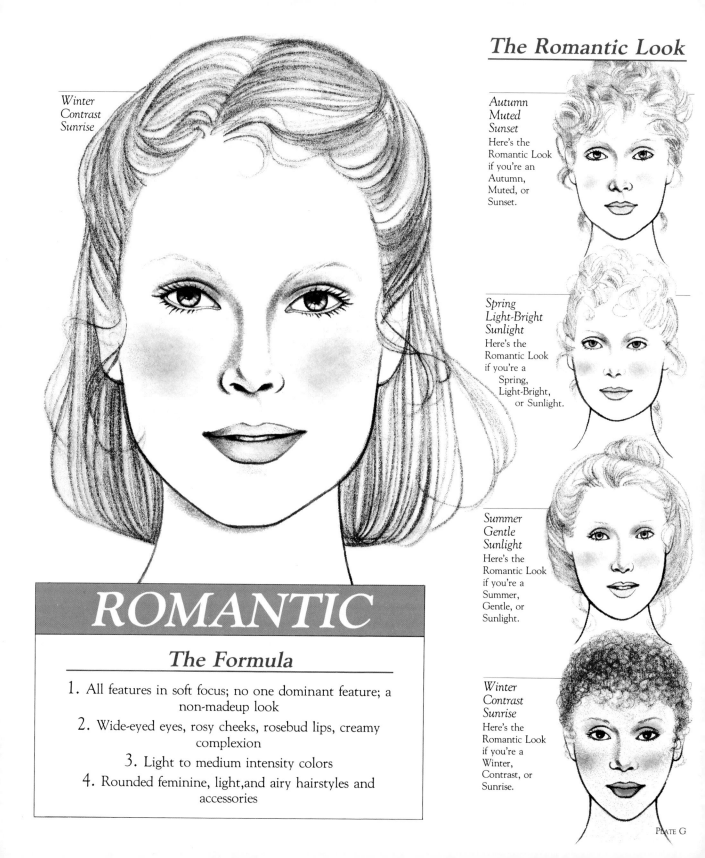

Winter Contrast Sunrise

The Romantic Look

Autumn Muted Sunset
Here's the Romantic Look if you're an Autumn, Muted, or Sunset.

Spring Light-Bright Sunlight
Here's the Romantic Look if you're a Spring, Light-Bright, or Sunlight.

Summer Gentle Sunlight
Here's the Romantic Look if you're a Summer, Gentle, or Sunlight.

Winter Contrast Sunrise
Here's the Romantic Look if you're a Winter, Contrast, or Sunrise.

ROMANTIC

The Formula

1. All features in soft focus; no one dominant feature; a non-madeup look
2. Wide-eyed eyes, rosy cheeks, rosebud lips, creamy complexion
3. Light to medium intensity colors
4. Rounded feminine, light, and airy hairstyles and accessories

The Earthy Palette

Your best Earthy colors are neutral, warm, and are of medium to dark intensity. They're generally opaque, not sheer or shimmery.

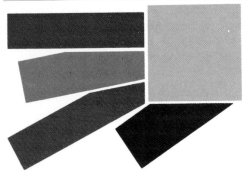

Autumn
Muted
Sunset

If your color key is Autumn, Muted, or Sunset, here are some of your Earthy colors:

- olive green
- copper brown
- bronzed mustard
- burnt sienna
- deep chocolate

Spring
Light-Bright
Sunlight

If your color key is Spring, Light-Bright, or Sunlight, here are some of your Earthy colors:

- yellowed grey
- bright golden brown
- apricot parfait
- sunny bright yellow
- ripe peach

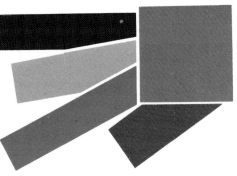

Summer
Gentle
Sunlight

If your color key is Summer, Gentle, or Sunlight, here are some of your Earthy colors:

- rosewood
- dusty mauve
- pink cocoa
- slate blue
- rosy brown

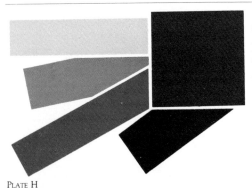

Winter
Contrast
Sunrise

If your color key is Winter, Contrast, or Sunrise, here are some of your Earthy colors:

- royal purple
- smoke grey
- flannel grey
- charcoal grey
- deep royal navy

The Earthy Image

Earthy is casual, wholesome, sensual, healthy, and sun-touched.

Earthy hair can be frizzy, wispy, untamed, layered, and windblown. It's length can be short, medium, or long.

Earthy jewelry and accessories are dangly, made of natural materials, and loose.

Earthy clothing is casual, loose, non-traditional, and non-dramatic.

Step-by-Step

The Goal: eyebrow and eye emphasis, natural face

Complexion

1. Cover blemishes only — not freckles — with medium tone concealer
2. If you need foundation, just barely apply a warm color with a sponge

Face Color

3. Copy the sun's kiss: cheek to cheek across the nose using creme, gel, or liquid color
4. Lightly sun kiss either the temples or just above the eyebrow, or the forehead, nose, and chin

Eyebrows

5. Use brow brush to brush hairs straight up for an unruly appearance
6. Use brow powder to darken a straight line across the underbrow skin (to camouflage arch and darken and thicken brow)

Eyes

7. Dust with smokey, earth tone shadow from lash to brow
8. Mascara the lashes: a little for carefree, more heavily for exotic

Lips

9. Touch with gloss for carefree, or line lip edges with neutral pencil for exotic

Illustrations by Christine Turner

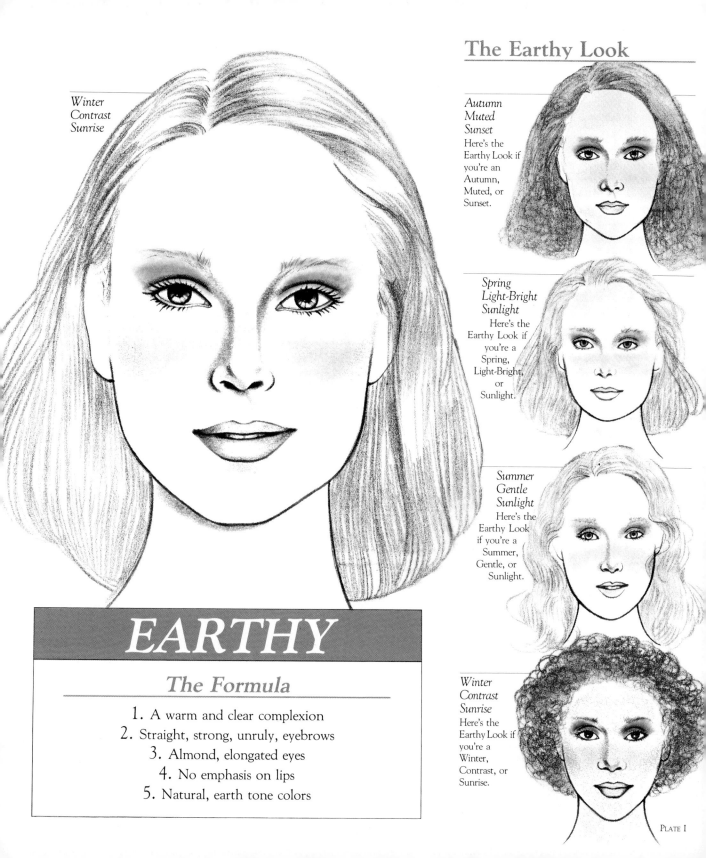

*Winter
Contrast
Sunrise*

The Earthy Look

*Autumn
Muted
Sunset*
Here's the
Earthy Look if
you're an
Autumn,
Muted, or
Sunset.

*Spring
Light-Bright
Sunlight*
Here's the
Earthy Look if
you're a
Spring,
Light-Bright,
or
Sunlight.

*Summer
Gentle
Sunlight*
Here's the
Earthy Look
if you're a
Summer,
Gentle, or
Sunlight.

*Winter
Contrast
Sunrise*
Here's the
Earthy Look if
you're a
Winter,
Contrast, or
Sunrise.

EARTHY

The Formula

1. A warm and clear complexion
2. Straight, strong, unruly, eyebrows
3. Almond, elongated eyes
4. No emphasis on lips
5. Natural, earth tone colors

PLATE I

The Glamour Palette

Your best Glamour colors are very light or very dark. They may be sheer, shiny or vivid. Glamour colors are always very intense.

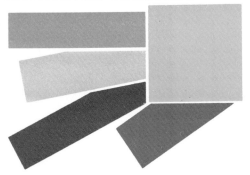

Autumn
Muted
Sunset

If your color key is Autumn, Muted, or Sunset, some of your Glamour colors are:
- hot brandied apricot
- antique deep turquoise
- smokey chartreuse
- bordeaux plum
- red orange heat

Spring
Bright-Light
Sunlight

If your color key is Spring, Bright-Light, or Sunlight, some of your Glamour colors are:
- flame
- hot violet
- bright buttercream
- popsicle orange
- bright aqua

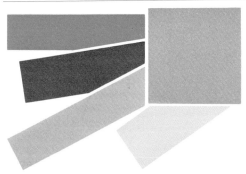

Summer
Gentle
Sunlight

If your color key is Summer, Gentle, or Sunlight, some of your Glamour colors are:
- vivid sky
- darkest blue cornflower
- deep watermelon
- hot lavender
- opal aqua

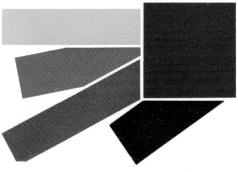

Winter
Contrast
Sunrise

If your color key is Winter, Contrast, or Sunrise, some of your Glamour colors are:
- magenta
- hot turquoise
- fuchsia bright
- hot purple
- midnight ebony

The Glamour Image

Glamour is dramatic, vivid, dazzling, bold, and sophisticated.

Glamour hair is angular, exaggerated, and high volume. It can be curled or sleek and severe. And it can be short, medium, or long in length.

Glamour jewelry and accessories are large, trendy, stark, angular. They're often plastic, metal, sparkly, wooden, or glass.

Glamour clothing is sophisticated, avant-garde, sexy, extreme, and high fashion.

Step-by-Step

The Goal: complexion, eye, and lip emphasis

Complexion
1. Quickly perfect it: cover circles, blemishes with light color concealer
2. Apply light color foundation with sponge

Cheekbones
3. Add slight amount of color, from hairline to no closer than outer rim of colored iris of eye

Eyes
4. Line upper and lower eyelids with crayon or pencil
5. Line crease of eye with shadow, crayon, or pencil
6. Dust on eye shadow
7. Coat lashes with mascara

Lips
8. Line lips with pencil
9. Add lip color and high gloss

Finishing Touches
10. Dust face with powder: translucent, pearlized, or translucent/pearlized mixture

Illustrations by Christine Turner

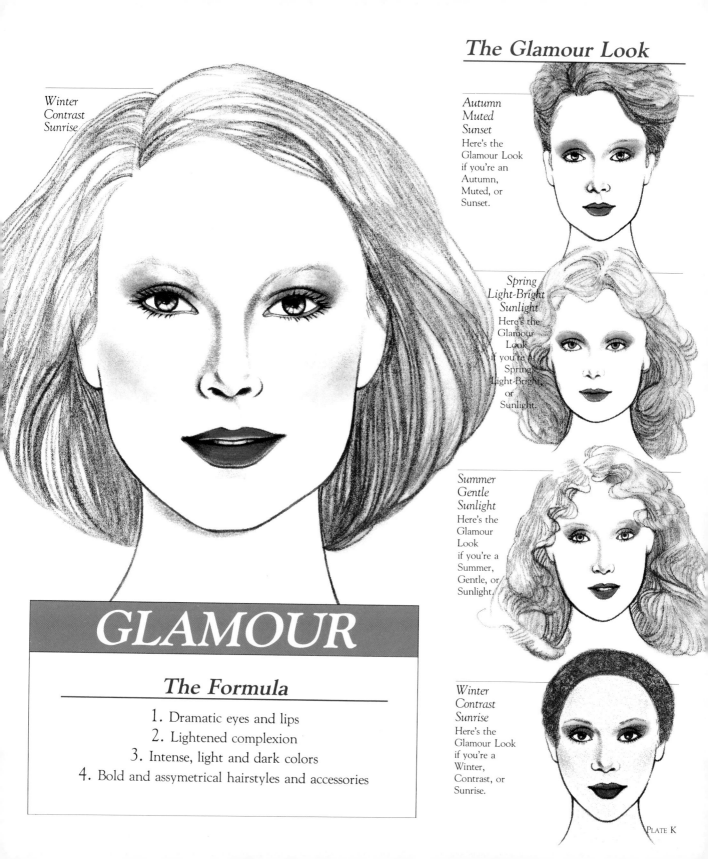

Winter
Contrast
Sunrise

The Glamour Look

Autumn
Muted
Sunset
Here's the
Glamour Look
if you're an
Autumn,
Muted, or
Sunset.

Spring
Light-Bright
Sunlight
Here's the
Glamour
Look
if you're a
Spring,
Light-Bright,
or
Sunlight.

Summer
Gentle
Sunlight
Here's the
Glamour
Look
if you're a
Summer,
Gentle, or
Sunlight.

Winter
Contrast
Sunrise
Here's the
Glamour Look
if you're a
Winter,
Contrast, or
Sunrise.

GLAMOUR

The Formula

1. Dramatic eyes and lips
2. Lightened complexion
3. Intense, light and dark colors
4. Bold and assymetrical hairstyles and accessories

PLATE K

Contouring Can Improve Your Look

Contouring with makeup is an easy way to beautify your face. Contouring can visually correct flaws in your face shape and features and make them conform to our current standard of beauty.

Lights and shadows are used in contouring. Lights are used on features to bring them forward, make them narrow, and make them angular. Shadows are used on features to make them recede, look larger, and look hollow.

Here are a few contouring techniques you'll want to try. Turn to Chapter 9 to learn how to fit them into the guidelines for each Image. In Chapter 9 you'll also find many other contouring tricks.

Eye-Brightening Blush

This technique intensifies eye color and adds a glow to your face. Place thin line of rouge or lipstick on orbital bone, parallel from brow arch to brow end. Blend lightly.

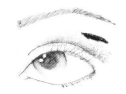

The Ideal Eye

When the eyes are open in a natural manner, an eye would fit in the distance between the lash line and the underside of the eyebrow. The distance between the two eyes is the length of one eye. Compare this illustration with your own eyes.

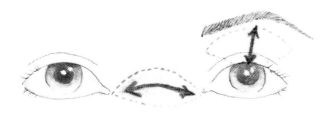

Wide-Set Eyes

Keep eyelids dark, with inner half of crease strongly defined. Eyeliner is widest at inner eye and tapers out to outer corner. Put dark shadow on inner half of lids and lighten it toward outer half. Begin eyebrows closer to nose than tear duct. Concentrate mascara on inner lashes.

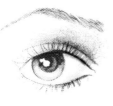
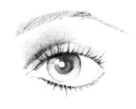

Eye-Opener Iris Dots

For a wide-eyed look, place one dot of light color on center of each eyelid, practically in lashes. Blur edges slightly.

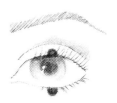

Close-Set Eyes

Eye makeup begins slightly toward center of eyelid from tear duct. Shadow starts light at inner third of lid and darkens gradually toward outer third. Highlight the triangle from tear duct to highest point of brow arch. Concentrate mascara on outer lashes.

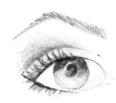
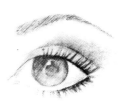

Deep-Set Eyes

Bring eyelid forward with lights and emphasize crease with darker color. Highlight under entire length of eyebrow. Line lower lashes, extending line beyond corner of eye. Use lots of mascara.

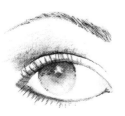
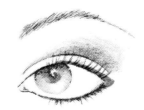

Duel-Eyeliner Technique

For extra eye drama, apply liquid eyeliner into lashes on top and bottom lids. Smudge with swab or pencil liner. Next, line both lids in normal fashion with pencil or powder and blur so liquid liner makes lash line look very full.

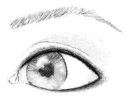

PLATE L

Necklines and Collars

Lace, ruff, or ruffle collars are romantic; so are sweetheart-shaped and Regency-scoop necklines. High-button front or shirtwaist style are demurely romantic. Ribbons threaded through lace or tatting are a pretty touch for either necklines or collars.

Some Favorite Fabrics

Organdy, organza, crepe, crepe de chine, chiffon, net, satin combined with other textures—like lace, water-marked or regular taffeta, grosgrain, velvet, georgette, lace, silk, cotton batiste, gauze, and other such fabrics are usually romantic in feeling. Lambswool and angora in delicate styles can also look romantic.

Special Accessories

- Round, old-fashioned wire-rim glasses
- Pearls, cameos, small cloisonne', mille fiori, or porcelain jewelry
- Reticules and other small purses
- Dressy, dainty sandal heels, "ballet" slippers, and bedroom slippers with eyelet, ribbon, lace

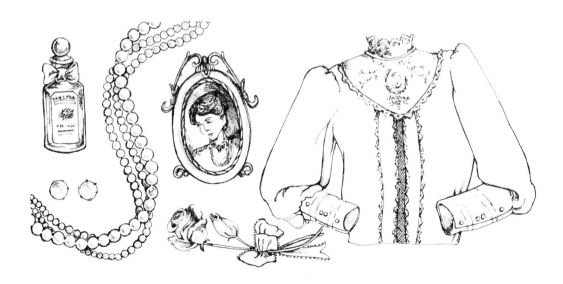

Romantic Magic by Candlelight

Romance and candlelight are a perfect match, aren't they? The mellow ambiance of candlelight is like old lace or aged wine, and Romantic Face fits right in. It might fade away at a discotheque but it has an innocent allure all its own at a dimly lit dinner for two!

The pearlized powder tips are found in the special section in this book for "After-5:00" techniques. They are lovely for Romantic Image because they suggest a dewy skin shimmer. Try a violet, lavender, aubergine, or purple highlighter in the deep crease of the eyelid. Follow the tips on pink touches in that special section especially closely, for they suit Romantic very well.

Your lips and cheeks may be a hint more colorful than you would wear in the daytime Romantic formula. Stay in the formula, but use a heavier hand, for your light Romantic looks can fade if you apply your evening makeup to suit your home mirror instead of night-lights elsewhere.

You may even want to add a few individual, varied-color artificial lashes to top and bottom eyelids—in the center only—for an exceptionally large, round, starry-eyed look for evening. See Model Face—Glamour Image for complete instructions, if you need them, on artificial eyelashes application.

Turn to the Candlelight basics chapter to learn more about after 5:00 techniques. Add pearls and swirls, and capture the dreamiest of evenings!

My Romantic Model Face

What Do I Need to Know Before I Begin?

Your creamiest complexion is vital to this look; use products that give you the sheerest possible appearance. A light moisturizer underneath your makeup will give you a dewy surface—neither oily, shiny, nor dry.

Your foundation should contain as much "white tone" as you can wear. Choose a color that you can describe as "fair" for you. Lightest translucent powder can be used to give a flawless look instead of great quantities of foundation. Be sure to use light concealer on flaws. Matte powder will finish this complexion.

Under-base tint. Apply a sheer film of under-base tint for skin coverage and color-correction/lightening under foundation. Choose the lightest, whitest variety you can wear. This can be a very soft, creamy, easy to blend coverage product—a whitish, sheer foundation that is a few shades lighter than your own skin tones—or an under-base product designed for this purpose. Use a sponge to blend it over your face. This creates the fine-textured, flawless Romantic complexion and reduces the amount of makeup you need to design this face.

Foundation. Keep it as light in color and as sheer in application as possible. If you've used an under-base tint, thinly spreading your foundation will be easy and speedy.

Choose a color containing white tones, and as fair as you can wear well—usually two shades lighter than your skin tones. Colors with the word "ivory" in the name are generally wonderful for naturally pale skins. Step up to a beige with a high "white" content if your skin tones are darker (look for words like "bisque"). Be sure to choose blue-based or yellow-based according to your own coloring.

Instead of ivories and light, white skin tones for foundations, concealers, and under-base tints (your complexion products), dark-skinned or golden-skinned romantics will choose creamy tones that develop a smooth, pale-for-you, skin surface.

Any skin color may use a foundation product with a "rose or pink" cast very effectively for Romantic Face. Choose cool ones if you're blue-based, and warm ones if you're yellow-based. However, those with yellow-based coloring should avoid foundation colors containing the words "golden, warm, copper, bronze, or honey." They're usually more yellow than Romantic look requires.

Compare several colors and then choose the optimum. With your flawless veneer in place, you're ready to add the pastel colorings.

Rosy cheeks, or peaches-and-cream complexion, characterize Romantic Face. The old-fashioned "apple-cheek" method of applying rouge on the high points of the cheekbones, toward the center of the face, creates a lovely natural-blush illusion for your Romantic Face.

It's easy to do—just think of Raggedy Ann—but then blend! Keep in a small circular area when blending, so it doesn't end up all over your cheeks. The more generously you apply it and thoroughly blend it in, the more it will look like your natural flush.

Always use a creme rouge. A gel would be your second choice, and powder blushers should not be used on the cheeks of your Romantic Face. No other products create the same dewy flush that a creme does. Are you concerned that rouge is heavy and "old-fashioned"? It looks startlingly strong in the compact but once blended with a sponge, it actually looks more natural than any other blush product! It just needs a little blending.

Even those with oily skins should use the creme rouge, a color stick, or a creme compact. You require more touch-up than your dry-skinned counterpart, because your makeup rises up on the oil and tends to slide off. The advantage is that your creme rouge goes on more easily, over your moist skin, and looks more natural.

The deepest part of the rouge color should be under the pupil of the eye. Don't bring the rouge lower than about the lobe of the ear.

If your face is classified as a round shape (see the contouring chapter), you'll need a small amount of contouring in addition to your rouge. Use a gentle, light shade of a dry powder blush or contour product—a medium shade, in a non-frosted coral, rose, or red powder, for example (depending upon your natural coloring).

Suck in your cheeks: the hollow created under your cheekbones, which runs from earlobe to the corner of the lips, is the trail you will dust with the blusher to contour.

Keep it light, so that the finished look is soft and does not create a visable angle—rather a soft shadow to compensate for the rounded blush shape being repeated onto your rounded facial shape. On a round face, you bring the contour powder—especially a light-colored one—down from the center of the ear all the way to the corner of the lip, if it looks good.

Eyebrows. Natural, soft curves characterize every feature of this image; your brows are no exception. If your brows are a medium-to-dark color, simply brush them in a natural curve, rounding them as much as you can to diminish any angular arching. Fair brows may need a little color, but try special, very light colors like blonde, gold, and palest brown shades.

Don't let the brows dominate the face. If you have classic brows in a medium-to-dark color, just smear some under-base color with your fingers through the brow, and let the spikiness go unsmoothed.

Some very dark brows are best lightened (with bleach, perhaps) if your job or lifestyle allows you to sustain a Romantic Image as your primary face. Otherwise, removing any stray hairs with tweezers or cuticle scissors and then dusting your brows with light or pearlized powder should help. Or you may smudge in some under-base tint. Don't brush the powder out afterward.

Eye makeup is fast and easy to apply with hints of color and rounded, dusky lids. The pastel colors, smoky and clear, are your top choices, as they assist in your desired "soft-focus" look.

Metallic and pearlized eye shadows detract from the aura; colors with a pink cast enhance. Aquas, turquoise, and light greens and purples are the ideal; earth tones and strong primary colors are too demanding for this image.

Dark-skinned Romantics are the only complexion type that can utilize a dusty charcoal, grey-green taupe, or rosy coffee as their darkest color. When choosing eye shadow or crayon for the eyelid, you still utilize a wide stroke with a doming emphasis over the center. You may apply shadows in any method, of course, that creates a rounded innocence.

Choose two colors, one a darker, more neutral shade. Crayons or powders are best for the darker shade; powder eye shadows or blushers, or soft creams, are best for the lighter color. The darker color is for the eyeliner. The lighter color is for above.

Mascara. You may leave it off, or use the lightest of colors—light browns and pastels are lovely—in small amounts. Mascara or heavy lashes create Classic, Earthy, and Glamour eyes. For Romantic Face, use a hint, concentrating it on the center lashes, rather than evenly across, for the open-eyed, starry-eyed look of the romantic. Curl your lashes, if you like.

Since you seldom color the under-eyelid, the barest hint of mascara on lower lashes can look especially good if your upper lashes have no added color. Detectable artificial lashes for daywear Romantic are not acceptable; a few individual, brown lashes at night may work if you're very handy with them.

Lips. Like eye shadows, lip color should be pastel, non-metallic, non-vivid, and light-to-medium in color. Apply a sheer lip color in the pinkest tint that becomes you—choose from medium rose, plum, carnation, pinky-coral, peach or salmon. Heavy gloss destroys the "soft-focus" impact, as do frosted and vibrant colors. Use a lip brush, but not a sharp lipliner pencil unless it is a lip gloss pencil.

A final note for dark-skinned Romantics: blue-based brown and black complexions should stay with pink undertones and colors for lipstick, rouge, eye shadow, and foundation. Yellow-based skins are best in peach, apricot, and warm undertones and colors.

The Romantic Bride

The Romantic Image is made for brides, especially when your fiance is the type who "hates makeup!"

Be sure you've tried this image out before the big day; the time to shock your groom is not when he sees you at the altar. Dress rehearsals are a good idea for everything, including your face. Your groom wants a familiar as well as glowing face on the vision walking up to him, and you want to be familiar with your Romantic Image so that it does look natural and like YOU!

Consider Your Bridal Photography

Since the makeup for your Romantic Face is soft and subtle, be sure to check with your photographer about film and lighting to augment your coloring. If you're yellow-based, make sure his lighting and film are not designed to best complement blue-based backgrounds and skin tones. Ask to see samples of his work.

Spend a little more time applying your face, especially with under-base tint, which is essential. If you lack cheek color, add extra; it will fade with the heat of the excitement. By adding extra color to every feature (so no one feature is more dominant than your cheeks), you can "tone up" the makeup a little for the camera. Heavier lip gloss can be used for your photography, although lip color should remain pastel or light.

Consider Your Bridal Accessories

There are many available accessories for wedding gowns. Perhaps you even have some family heirlooms, or some traditional customs, that you'd like to include in your plan. Are they romantic in feeling, to match your total look?

Some romantic accessories are:
- Juliet cap, with seed pearls
- Flower wreath, fresh or dried
- Antique combs for ornate hairstyle or cathedral veil (or antique-look, such as ivory or tortoise shell with gold trim)
- Lace, Lace, Lace

- Tiny pearl buttons buttoning up the back of your gloves or your dress
- Sweetheart neckline, especially with scallops of lace
- Tiny pearl earrings, necklace, bracelet, garter
- Fingernails: pale, rounded tips, no talons, moons may show
- Fragrance: sweet, light, feminine; possibly fruity, floral, or lightly spicy like potpourri

Romantic Model Face: Tool Checklist

Cosmetic Products

☐ Sheer moisturizer
☐ Under-base tint
☐ Foundation/Makeup Base
   —sheerest, creamiest possible
   —lightest color you can wear (2 shades lighter than skin tone) with
     large percentage of white in it
☐ Translucent Powder (light color)
☐ Creme Rouge, Creme Rouge Stick, or Creme Color Compact
   —pink-tone cast, non-shimmer
☐ Lip Balm
   —very sheer, low gloss
   —pink-tone cast
☐ Lipstick
   —light-to-medium, sheer color
   —opaque, non-frosted, not vibrant
☐ Eye Crayon or Powder Eyeliner, and an Eye Shadow
   —pastel, clear, or muted
   —opaque, soft neutral
   —best colors for either: green or purple family
☐ Mascara
   —very light colors: brown or pastels

Cosmetic Tools

☐ Makeup "silk" sponge
☐ Powder complexion brush and powder pad
☐ Eyebrow brush
☐ Natural sea sponge
☐ Lipstick brush

Model Face—Romantic Formula

Glowing Complexion; All Features Equal Emphasis

1. Romantic Complexion

Smooth on under-base tint thinly, with sponge, to level and color-correct, including brows if desired.

With your very light cover product, give blemishes, under-shadows, veins, liver spots, and freckles a casual coverage. Add any special contouring you need to reduce any dominant facial features.

Spread foundation sparingly with makeup sponge, avoiding eye area but covering lips. The correct light color won't need to reach to the hairline.

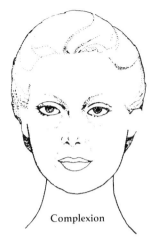

Complexion

2. Romantic Cheeks

To rouge cheeks, first smile broadly, theatrically. Rouge the round "apples" of flesh that appear under the outside corner of the eye, on top of your cheekbones.

Don't apply rouge above or to the under-sides of the apples. And bring it no closer to your nose than the pupil of your eye. Blend well with makeup sponge; keep rouge contained in the small "apple" areas.

Dust face lightly with translucent powder, using pad or complexion brush. Powder is very light on the apples.

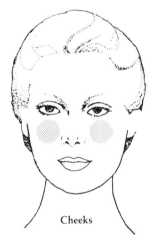

Cheeks

3. Romantic Eyes

Brush brows to rounded shape. Then smooth on light face powder with your pad to lighten and soften, unless you have extremely light brows or have used under-base tint already.

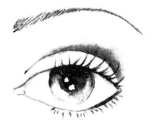

Rounded Brow

The
Romantic
Face

Softly line the upper eyelid with the darker crayon, using a wide stroke. Make the section of the eye shadow over the pupil (center part of the eye) considerably wider so that the liner "domes." Curve it around the outer corner of the eye; this helps "cut" the angle and diminish any slant.

Now add the lighter color gently to the crease, wider near the inner corner if that becomes you. You may also carry it up a little beyond the crease, onto the underside of the orbital (brow) bone. Blend and smooth.

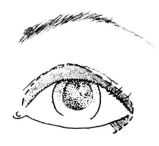

Horizontal Eye Makeup/Rounded

4. Romantic Lips

Lips are already covered with foundation. If you wish to use a lip pencil, it should be blunt, not sharp, and used on its side rather than its point. Outline your lips widely, with a mere hint of color.

Apply a sheer lip gloss with a brush, and blend pencil and gloss to create a natural rosebud lip.

Add sheer lip color.

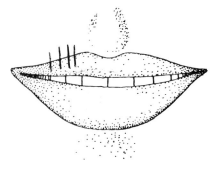

Lips

5. Finishing Touches

Pat face with sea sponge that has been thoroughly wetted and then squeezed "dry." This adds a natural and dewy, moist look, with the added benefit of "setting" the makeup to last.

Add 2 or 3 individual lashes to the center of the top and bottom eyelids, for a "starry-eyed" look, if you feel it's needed.

Mascara the lashes, lightly, concentrating on the center lashes to maintain the rounded, eye shape.

Now that you're looking and feeling deliciously feminine, turn back to the Check-Out, earlier in this Romantic chapter, to be sure you've got the formula right.

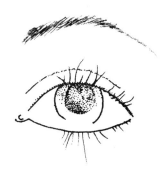

"Starry-Eyed" Mascara

Chapter 4

The Glamour Face

Setting the Mood

From the earliest days of cosmetics, this face has been the First Lady of beauty. Royalty has often used this image to project a larger-than-life quality, from Egypt's Nefertiti and Cleopatra to today's own Princess Diana.

Its mood is excitement, dash, and pizazz. Almost everything goes, and glamour enjoys setting trends for makeup, hair and fashion. Most accessories and clothes are designed for this image; it's the daring darling of the beauty industry.

Glamour laughs at itself, loves its own flair, and adores making its own trends obsolete almost before they've caught on. Every flight of fantasy can be indulged for a moment, or distilled and re-introduced time and time again.

It's confident, supple, sparkling, sexy, and sometimes a little frivolous. Its image is drama, chic, color, and style, from the classy revered Chanel look to the avant-garde or even bizarre.

Everyone gets a lift from it, and you will, too, especially from the entertainment its endless variety provides.

How Did Glamour Image Become so Popular?

Glamour has always been popular. For centuries, glamour was reserved for the leisure classes, who had time and servants to apply cosmetics, and the affluence to purchase jewels, precious metals, and prized fabrics. The leaders of glamour have always set the fashion pace of the innovative and untried.

Walter Raleigh's Queen Elizabeth more likely used arsenic for her white face, and Japanese Kabuki makeup still influences modern makeup products. Egyptian kohl-eyes are much copied today. And Scarlett O'Hara didn't bite her lips to turn them pale!

The basic formula for glamour beauty today has not changed since the days of Nefertiti; only cosmetic tools and fashions have changed.

Famous Glamour Faces

Long ago queens—Cleopatra, Nefertiti, Elizabeth I, Snow White's mother—wore Glamour. Cinema queens—Gloria Swanson, Marlene Dietrich, Greta Garbo—knew a good thing to copy when they saw it.

Modern celebrities know that glamour is the image that shines best from afar, so it is the choice of those who are constantly in the public eye. Famous names of recent vintage who have favored glamour are: Rita Hayworth, Marilyn Monroe, Diana Ross, Cher, Lucille Ball, Dolly Parton, Sally Struthers, Gloria Vanderbilt, Marisa Berenson, Shirley MacLaine, Ann-Margret, and Marie Osmond.

Softer glamour figure are: Peggy Lee, Zsa Zsa and Eva Gabor, Arlene Dahl, Julie Andrews, Stephanie Powers, Shirley Jones and Barbara Cartland.

Rive Gauche glamour figures are: Shari Belafonte, Margaux Hemingway, the "Charlie" girl, and Sheena Easton.

Princess Diana trend-sets a classy style of glamour all her own.

Why and When Do You Wear the Glamour Image?

The first place to turn, when you want an aura of up-to-the-minute chic, is to your Glamour Image. In addition to impressing everyone in the vicinity that you are not behind the times, you set a mood of excitement.

Do you want sexy but not earthy, or eye-catching but not authoritative? Do you feel confident and amusing? Glamour image is all those, plus it can add maturity to the baby-faced, or an attractive sense of high-spirited agelessness to the maturing woman.

Glamour Face draws attention away from flaws, and accents the features that are usually a woman's most flattering and dramatically feminine: eyes, lips, and complexion. It can be used to grab the eye distractingly.

This is the most appropriate image to complement strikingly colored hair, or very severe, high-fashion hairstyles.

Glamour Face is the perfect face to top whatever is the latest in fashion and style trends. In fact, your choice of garment may indisputably determine that Glamour is the face to wear with it. If you've just bought something trendy, sophisticated, or dramatically cut, you'll need a face that is in sync with the mood of the garment—and Glamour is the one.

The suggestion of worldly sophistication clings to this face. Doesn't every woman want to evoke such an impression at some time? When you do need to look most sophisticated, choose Glamour.

Need I add that Glamour Image is not for: a first impression in a difficult setting, conservative or career environs, or for your mud-wrestling or shy violet impulses?

Nor is it appropriate on young teenagers, whose just-budding glow conflicts with the full-blown worldliness of the look.

Where Do You Wear the Glamour Image?

Glamour is the single most popular image for evenings out. It creates sparkle and attracts men. Although it is the image most suited to evening occasions and lighting, it is not necessarily limited to after 5:00.

Your career may require a look of high-fashion if it is in the world of modeling, cosmetology, the fashion/beauty industry, photography, the arts, advertising, acting, contemporary music, dance, or other entertainment endeavors. If you're not in the business, but like to attend theatre, ballet, opera, and other dramatic arts, use their inspiration for your own—your Glamour Face.

Any time you want to make a splash for entertaining, get-togethers, parties, reunions, dates, dinners, and possibly conventions, add pizazz with your Glamour artistry.

Stimulating haunts like jazz clubs, discos, concerts, and private clubs are a showcase for your Glamour choices.

Or perhaps you're just going shopping or to an event where everyone looks exciting but you. Whether you're on a daytime or evening outing, Glamour

Image keeps you from fading into the woodwork or feeling lost in the shade of someone else's drama.

What are the Characteristics of the Glamour Face

The key to the Glamour Image is drama of every kind, but always with the understanding that you will accent some of your best features and stay within the Glamour formula.

The Glamour formula is simply:

- Deep, brilliant, large eyes
- Glossy, outstanding, often colorful lips
- Unflawed-looking, pale skin
- Vivid, intense or unusual colors
- Dramatic styles

Any face shape will work. Angular features and high cheekbones have the most drama, but they aren't necessary. Just be sure to bring out those eyes and lips with makeup.

Introducing You to the Glamour Image Formula

Do I Have Time for It?

If you'd like a jazzy face, and there's room in your life for chic, you'll have time for a Glamour face. You can wear a fast-and-easy version or spend hours on this image.

If this is your favorite face for painting yourself and the town "pink," and you include bubble baths, manicures, pedicures, perfume pyramid, and picture-perfect glamour hair, you can really while away an hour just getting into the glamour mood! When these rituals add to your enjoyment, and aura, you may not want to count the time cost either.

But because "anything goes" for Glamour, you can dramatize those features required by the Fast Face formula and run out the door. You really can pull together a glamour look in 8 minutes or less. Like all the other images, the keystone is the balance of power of the features, styling of accessories, and choices of color and line.

If time is of the essence, stick to the Fast Face, and 8-minute glamour will be your reward.

Glamour Fast Face

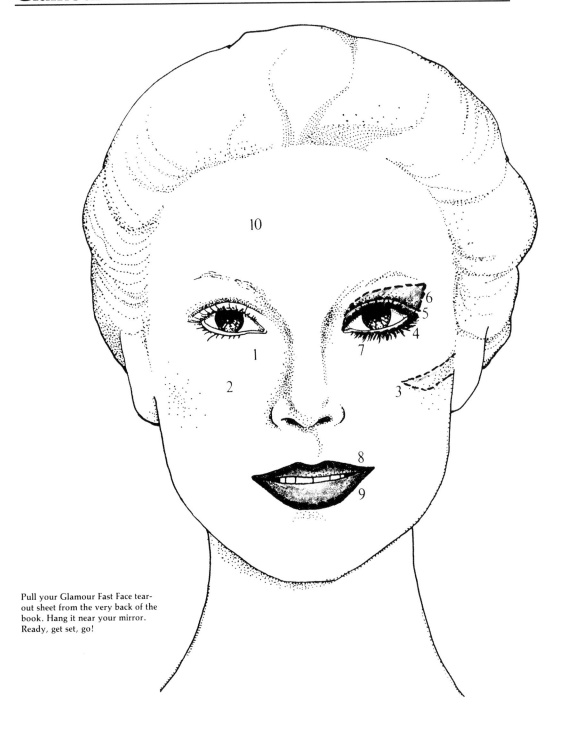

Pull your Glamour Fast Face tear-out sheet from the very back of the book. Hang it near your mirror. Ready, get set, go!

Ready To Try Glamour Face?

Whether you use the Fast Face or the Model Face makeover, the more closely you follow this glamour-appeal code, the greater the reactions you will evoke with your exciting new face.

—Fast Face—Glamour Formula

Complexion, Eyes, Lips

Complexion

1 Quickly perfect it: cover circles, blemishes with light-color concealer
2 Apply light-color foundation with makeup sponge

Cheekbones

3 Add slight amount of color, from hairline to no closer than outer rim of colored iris of eye

Eyes

4 Line upper and lower eyelids with crayon or pencil
5 Line crease of eye with shadow, crayon, or pencil
6 Dust on eye shadow
7 Coat lashes with mascara

Lips

8 Line lips with pencil
9 Add lip color and high gloss

Finishing Touches

10 Dust face with powder: translucent, pearlized, or translucent/pearlized mixture
   • Be sure no "L.O.T" (lipstick on teeth)!

Does Glamour Work on Me?

This face is the ultimate in flexibility! Every skin type, coloring, shape, and age can enjoy this face, except the very young. It has few restrictions, and it can work around your best and worst features. Overtly sexy and sophisticated, it always produces exciting elan.

Everybody has eyes and lips they can accentuate. Also, the less sun-drenched the skin appears, the greater the glamour look.

If your eyes and lips are strong features that demand attention naturally, it will be especially simple for you to acquire a Glamour Face. It may become your number-1 favorite.

To summarize the basics for creating your Glamour Face:

- Complexion: your palest, most creamy; either matte or iridescent.
- Eyes: horizontal or vertical makeup lines, focal point equal to lips; deep, brilliant, large, compelling, often shimmery.
- Lips: full, outstanding, glossy, often pouty; focal point equal to eyes; dramatically colorful or frosted.
- Eyebrows: any kind, as long as they don't dominate the eyes; a winged brow is very good, or a rounded brow for soft glamour.
- Colors: Brilliant, bold, vivid, intense, sharp, either opaque or shiny, extremes of dark or light.

A word of caution: Don't get carried so away with your makeup that you add it where it isn't needed—such as bright cheek color or straight, strong eyebrows—straying from the Glamour Face formula. You will look both over-madeup and image-less. That gives Glamour a bad name!

Your choice of colors and hairstyle can create a mood of drama, underscoring your face statement after your Glamour Face makeover. Jewelry, accessorizing, fragrance, and attitude add punch. Dress is chic.

The Total Look

Pulling It All Together

1. Creamy, perfect-looking skin characterizes Glamour Face: its color as light as possible for you, and usually in the beige or ivory families. All flaws should be visually corrected as much as possible. Complexion has either matte or pearlized finish.

2. The two most dominant features in the face are: eyes and lips. Eyes large and deep; lips noticeable or even pouty. Cheekbones may appear angular and high; eyebrows may appear winged or rounded.

3. Eyelids tend to be dramatized, lashes dramatic, and lips shiny or frosted. Almost everything goes.

4. Glamour is characterized by trendy, vivid, extreme, or smart colors, either opaque or iridescent. Glamour combines sexy with chic.

Eyebrows
1. Down-played, any shape
2. Winged is high glamour
3. Rounded is soft glamour
4. Straight is Rive Gauche glamour

Eyes
1. Maximize—accentuate to fullest
2. Horizontal or vertical makeup techniques
3. Plenty of lashes—fake, or heavily mascared real

Lips
1. Share limelight with eyes, equally
2. Stylized, "made-up," with lipliner
3. May be pouty
4. Vivid color; glossed or frosted

Complexion
1. Your palest
2. Creamy, flawless-looking
3. Matte or pearlized

Cheekbones
1. High, faintly glowing, and shimmery
2. May be sculpted, angular for dramatic glamour

Hair
1. Can be dramatic, angular cuts
2. Extreme (even slightly) styles
3. Can have dramatic coloring
4. Need not look natural
5. Hairstyle has flair

Ornaments
1. Sophisticated, trendy
2. Rarely tiny, diminutive, old
3. Exciting, pizazz
4. All textures, in mod style

Buzz Words
1. Eyes, lips
2. Intense or vivid colors
3. Iridescent shimmer
4. Drama, soft, or Rive Gauche
5. Charismatic, sleekly sexy
6. Sharp, smart, sophisticated
7. Drama, panache, chic, flair
8. Confident, exciting, extreme
9. Larger-than-life
10. Almost everything goes

Check It Out, And Go!

Is my foundation too dark?

Are my eyes and lips the first points of my face to be noticed?

Should I add any gloss, frost, or iridescence, or extra lashes?

Are my lipstick, nail polish, eye makeup colors too middle-of-the-road (medium) in intensity?

Do I sparkle? Does my fragrance?

Whatever your setting, enjoy your jewel-bright impact! You're gorgeous!

The Glamour Color Palette

Brilliant, sparkling, vivant—exciting colors create glamour. Shimmer and shine always say "pizazz."

Rather than medium shades and medium intensity, choose your very light and very dark colors to create interest and drama. The "coolest" colors that become you are best for Glamour Image. Any color can be glamorous, but those with sophistication are real impression-makers. Each color key offers some particularly glamorous colors.

Some Suggested Colors

Shocking pink	Tangy lemon yellow
Shocking red	Bright burgundy
Magenta	Hot tangerine
Fuchsia	Flame
Deep hot pink	Orange sherbet
Kelly green	Hot violet
Royal blue	Hot aqua
Peacock	Light-fire turquoise
Royal purple	Hot periwinkle blue
Garnet red	Clear, bright aqua
Platinum	
Brandied apricot	Cherry red
Golden coral	Rose-pink coral
Red penny	Cornflower blue
Bordeaux wine	Sky blue
Smoky magenta	Opal
Dark periwinkle blue	Creme de menthe
Deep teal	Hot orchid
Antique deep turquoise	Raspberry
Smoky turquoise	Abalone
Dusky lilac	Lacy blue agate
Celadon	Burnished plum
Chartreuse	Limeade
Gold lame	Rose pink
Watermelon	Blue-red
	Hot lavender

Glamour Sample Makeup Color Schemes

Fuchsia Bright Scheme

Concealer: Light/medium

Foundation: Cool beiges, ivories, or rachelles

Face Powder: Lightest translucent or pearlized

Highlighter: Light, pearlized

Creme Rouge: Fuchsia, or garnet

Powder Blush: With shimmer—magenta,or deep bright rose

Mascara: Midnight black, or any cold, royal colors

Eye Shadow: Royal purple or blue, silver, midnight blue, celestial blue
Frosts: blue, green, white

Lip Pencil: Shocking red, bright magenta, or fuchsia

Lipstick: With shimmer—shocking pink, fuchsia, magenta, or garnet

Hot Flame Scheme

Concealer: Light/medium

Foundation: Light ivories or beiges

Face Powder: Lightest translucent or pearlized

Highlighter: Pearlized butter cream

Creme Rouge: Flame, orange sherbet, or clear bright red

Powder Blush: With shimmer—hot red or clear coral

Mascara: Clear brown-black or clear warm green or aqua

Eye Shadow: Hot violet, hot aqua, light-fire turquoise, hot periwinkle blue, or clear bright aqua

Lip Pencil: Flame, hot coral, or orange sherbet

Lipstick: With heat, perhaps shimmer—orange sherbet, flame, hot red, or hot coral-pink

For the information of the serious color student:

*Clear, Cold, Blue-based
(Winter/Contrast/Sunrise)*

*Clear, Warm, Yellow-based
(Spring/Light-Bright/Sunlight)*

Sample Makeup Color Schemes

Mercurochrome Cherry Scheme

Concealer: Off-white

Foundation: Cool ivories, beiges as light as possible

Face Powder: Lightest translucent or pearlized

Highlighter: Off-white, pearlized

Creme Rouge: Hot rose; mercurochrome pink

Powder Blush: With shimmer watermelon; cherry red; or raspberry

Mascara: Soft black, or any hazy, cool color

Eye Shadow: [may shimmer] blue, opal, hot orchid, abalone, limeade, hot lavender, cornflower blue

Lip Pencil: Hot rose, bright pink, or watermelon

Lipstick: [may shimmer] watermelon, cherry red, or bright rose

Bronze Lamé Scheme

Concealer: Light as possible; 'oyster' family, or warm beige

Foundation: Ivories, cane, beige as light as possible

Face Powder: Lightest translucent or pearlized

Highlighter: With shimmer: gold lamé or bronze

Creme Rouge: Red penny, or hot tomato

Powder Blush: With shimmer-brick, tomato, or dusty coral

Mascara: Brown or brown-black

Eye Shadow: [may shimmer] Sky bronze, chartreuse, teal gold lamé, deep periwinkle, dusky lilac, smoky turquoise, brandied apricot

Lip Pencil: Red copper or tomato red

Lipstick: [may shimmer] Hot tomato or candied brick

For the information of the serious color student:

Cloudy, Cool, Blue-based
Summer/Gentle/Sunlight

Cloudy, Warm, Yellow-based
Autumn/Muted/Sunset

Glamour Hair

Isn't this great—you've guessed it again—anything goes! From cropped punk purple, to swirling long locks, any style with flair will make the statement you want.

This is the image for drama, so if you are mad for a new show-stealing haircut, top it off with Glamour Face artistry.

Textures

The less natural-looking the texture, the more glamorous it appears. Go super-slick, high-sheen, asymmetrical, or go fuzzy and wild. But don't go totally unstyled, that's Earthy.

Lengths

Any length can be exciting when the cut is clearly evident. Very long and very short hair have innate drama simply because they're extreme. Just ensure that the style is as great as the length.

Designs and Styles

Super slick is always glamorous. Loose, severe, sculptured, razor, angular, and asymmetrical designs can all have glamour appeal. Glamour hair best augments your image when it's vivid or exaggerated, styled with flair, even if it's just barely exaggerated.

For example, if for Classic you usually pull your hair to the nape of your neck a little loosely or teased at the crown for body, now slick it back to a tight chignon for Glamour. Maybe even add a spit curl or a bang angled down one cheek.

Take your consistent style, and exaggerate it slightly by adding volume or a slightly more dramatic wave or curl. Or perhaps employ a few sophisticated combs.

If you wear an afro, curl it tighter for your glamour moments. If your hair is back-combed, maybe a little teasing at the crown would create drama. Or try slicking down the sides with sculpting lotion.

Glamour Hair Variations

Parts

Side or center parts can spell Glamour, especially side parts just above the ears, or no part at all.

Curls

Bigger or tighter, try more curls than you usually wear. "Sculpt" hair with combs, sparkly barrettes, or protein sculpture lotion. Very short afros for black women are pure Glamour. For all women, each inch of extra length on a short "afro" type silhouette brings you closer to a medium length and the Classic—not Glamour—style.

Waves

Waves are usually combined with straight hair elsewhere on the head to create drama. For instance, you may have a chin-length cut with the chin-length bang on one side permed in deep waves. Or your hair may be smooth to the ear, breaking into deep waves below, to the shoulders. You've seen the look; these are just a few examples.

Upswept

Bouffant is always Glamour. Too soft and gentle looks romantic, but swept up and over or away on one side is exaggerated and highly glamorous.

Bangs

Exaggerate them, at least slightly, if they're cut Classic (curler, curling iron, blow dryer). Little short-cropped bangs that stop in the middle of the forehead are Glamour, as are exaggeratedly long or uneven bangs, or a bang worn on one side of the head only. (Glamour bangs don't flatter the mature.)

Pony-Puffs

A single knot, or "pony tail" (may be curled, braided, or wrapped) of hair caught up from an otherwise loose, free hair design projects an unexpected, teasing, Glamour impact. It is very pouty and "ingenue" because of its playful surprise element.

Avant Garde

All truly avant-garde styles are Glamour (unusual, trend-setting, dramatic, unconventional). An example is the bowl-on-the-top-of-the-head cut (a la Richard III).

Braids

Multiple, looping braids can be glamorous, as can a long, fat braid. Braids are usually best with Glamour hair ornaments or Glamour bangs.

Hair Colorings

Dramatically or obviously "man-made" hair colors always radiate Glamour. The high-shine that these chemical colorings can also add to the hair is Glamorous, too. Platinum blonde or silver, carroty or fiery red, and raven or cherry black hair exemplify this look. Color crayons, temporary rinses and streak sprays can add to Glamour mania.

Hair Ornaments

Many hair ornaments are designed for glamour. Bold and geometric patterns, sparkles, dramatizers, and trendy stylers can be found in barrettes, hairbands, and hair combs.

These hair accessories should be dramatic in color, design, and fabric: wide hairbands, hair scarves, and other hair coverings, including cloches and turbans.

Flowers if used in the hair are large or medium sized; they can be of any material.

Trims and jewelry can be woven through the hair to develop eye-catching appeal.

Dust hair glitter over your hair to add after-5:00 sparkle or a frivolous touch of glamour.

Hair bound in the back by nets is unconventional in the 1980's and therefore usually projects a soft type of glamour, especially when worn with clothing styles hinting at glamour couture of by-gone eras.

Accessorize Your Glamour Face

Earrings

- Large, rather than tiny and diminutive
- Stark, rather than "soft-focus"
- Bold, vivid, and dramatic colors, materials, and shapes
- Glittery, iridescent, and shiny earrings add sparkle to your look
- Over-sized earrings add drama
- Best size: medium to large
- Best shape: square, triangular, sharply angular, dangling, geometric, or large circles (not large hoops; they're Earthy Image)
- Best materials: plastic, acrylic, lucite, plain or beaten metals, glitter, sparkle, man-made/synthetics, wood, glass

Scarves

Anything bold can add a glamour touch: scarves twisted into a choke "necklace"; tied in an oversized sailor bow, looped around the neck with the ends dangling, tied in square knots around the neck, arrayed as ascots for tailored glamour, shawl-tied about the shoulders, fanning out, pleated scarves, and so forth.

Try wrapping your hair, turban style, in a wide scarf, or wrapping one about your waist.

Collars and Necklines

Add a large flower to a glamour neckline for extra fun. Here are some glamour necklines: wide scoop, narrow scoop, wide or narrow v-neck, mandarin collar, side-button front, stand-up collar, Chanel cut, jewel-neck, tuxedo lapel, dramatic cowl-neck, stand-up ruff, shawl collar, or bateau (boat-neck) collar.

Some Favorite Fabrics

Glamour fabrics are: lamé, satin, sequinned, "shot" silk, raw silk, nylon, rayon, pointelle, acrylic, terry cloth, velour, knit, polished cotton polyester, among others.

Nails

Try white polish; a pearlized top coat; decorating with flowers, rhinestones; moons or tips painted; unusual and dramatic colors; glitter, metallics, or frost; or dragon talons for something new with your Glamour nails.

Facial Decoration

Patches, beauty spots, facial painting, glitter, and other decorations are all glamour accents. Paint them near temptress eyes and mouth to accent your best feature of the Glamour Face.

Special Accessories

- dramatic, high-fad glasses (sun, plain lens, or prescription)
- rhinestones; glitter; silver, gold, or bronze
- very high-heeled shoes, mules with swansdown for the boudoir
- oversize handbags
- current, high fashion, or trendy fads

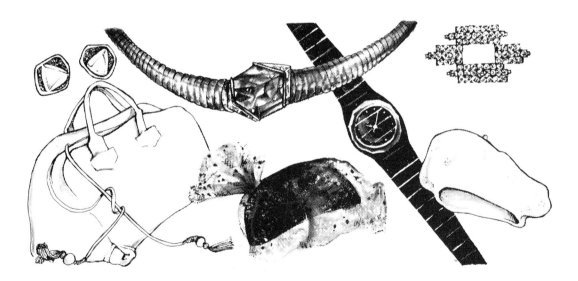

Glamour Magic by Candlelight

Glamour Face is almost everyone's favorite evening face. Why? You show up better at night in Glamour Face because it's strongly colorful and "made-up." Also, Glamour's dramatic nature suits the frequent drama of evening encounters. Daytime in Glamour Face spells pizazz, but your evening Glamour Image can be brilliantly effervescent!

Before you turn to the Candlelight Basics chapter, keep in mind that you're almost there already, in Glamour. In the Glamour formula, you're already emphasizing your lips and eyes, which are the best evening features to focus upon.

After 5:00 p.m., add extra mascara, additional lipstick and gloss, a hint more blusher if necessary, and more charcoal eye makeup. Be sure it's all in your coolest colors, even if it's cooler than your daytime choice.

And if you're really getting into the act, try a flicker of hair glitter, and a few false eyelashes if you don't already wear them regularly. Get as carried away with adding evening shimmer and naughty accessories as you like.

Check the Candlelight Basics chapter for further guidance.

My Glamour Model Face

What Do I Need to Know Before I Begin?

All styles of makeup application can be used in this face, as long as it follows the eye and lip emphasis formula. Careful blending isn't required; if you prefer a somewhat tailored sort of Glamour, you may blend, for a smoother look. Unblended, the ridges and edges of strong makeup application can enhance your most dramatic moods.

Foundation is best if it's a shade or two lighter than your natural skin tone, or a close match. The colors should be as "cool" as possible—not warm, sunny, honey, golden, tan, bronzy, or peachy. Stick with ivories, beiges, and rachelles.

Creamy-perfect skin is sophisticated and dramatic. You may want to use an under-base tint to establish the look of porcelain-perfect skin; crepey, more mature skin is especially enhanced by the technique. Crepey skins should also use colors more closely matching the skin tone, rather than lighter extremes.

To whiten skin for a truly dramatic, or Japanese "Kabuki" kind of look, generously apply a light-colored under-base tint, apply your lightest, sheerest foundation, and top it all off with a generously applied light or white powder. Additionally, use little or no cheek color, and use strong, dark eye and lip makeup.

Red, coral, or orange blusher between under-brow bone and eye crease intensifies the "Kabuki" (but not china doll) look.

Concealers can augment this Glamour Face by providing a creamy base for flaw coverage, and for smoothing over discolorations to promote that creamy finish. Choose a light color becoming to you.

Shimmery highlighter around the outer eye area calls attention to your lustrous eyes. Try an iridescent highlighter for maximum pizazz.

Translucent powder or pearlized, loose, face-finishing powder adds polish to your sophisticated look. Again, choose the lightest becoming shade. You may want to blend both plain and pearlized for your own shimmery finish. Use loose translucent powder for the best results.

Creme rouge applied the length of the cheekbone and near the outer corner of the eye creates a "flush." The less cheek color you wear, the greater the drama of your face. So you may want just a touch of creme rouge under your face powder and powder blush, or you can leave it off altogether.

Powder blushers are better than creme rouges because they are not as colorful and attention-grabbing. More subtle powder blushers can add a hint of color to the cheekbones, brightening the eyes and face without competing with the eye/lip emphasis. Powder blushers may also be used to sculpt high cheekbones by brushing in the hollows just underneath the cheekbone.

Shimmer and iridescent blushers provide sparkle. The more sparkle, the softer the Glamour look; the less sparkle (and more matte), the greater the drama.

Eyebrow art depends upon your mood. Keep eyebrow color light or to match your hair. Eyebrows are best when not emphasized as much as the eyes (and lips), although they may be made up somewhat, as part of the eye-area emphasis. Eyebrows more dominant than eyes tip the balance of power, resulting in neither Glamour nor Earthy Face.

Gently shape the brow, tweezing out the most unnecessary hairs on the brow bone above or below, following its natural lines, if Glamour is to be your everyday Face. You can vary your brow with your mood, making it straighter and stronger for stark Rive Gauche Glamour, or rounder and lighter for soft Glamour, or arching for a more tailored, classy Glamour.

One highly dramatic brow for your high-Glamour look is a winged brow, which tapers, lifting slightly, in a stylized manner out toward the hairline.

Lips are one of the two Glamour focal points. Lipliner may show, even demand attention, if you like. Lipliner should be sharp, and brilliant or dark. Frosted colors always project Glamour. Color may go outside the lip line if you like that look. The object of it all is a sophisticated, deliberately pouty lip! Heavy gloss suits this mood.

And finally we arrive at your gorgeous, Glamour eyes! As with lips, everything goes here, too. Vertical shadow techniques are highest Glamour. Eyeliner, iridescent and shimmer products, and lots of lashes are also great accents for your most dramatic eyes. Choose a technique that contours if there's something special you'd like to accomplish.

Crepey eyelid caution: matte shadows detract from crepiness; metallics emphasize crepiness. Use bright colors instead of shimmer.

Mascaras in glamour colors enhance your eye artistry.

Artificial lashes are a glamour statement. You may use either a strip, or band, or apply them individually for an unobtrusive statement if you will be seen close up. Here are instructions for both methods.

The strip, or band: Buy the varied-color-band type of lashes; human hair is considered best.

Holding the lashes in your hand or in their case with the fringe out, trim every third lash by hand with cuticle scissors to a natural-looking length close to that of your own natural lashes.

For a perfect lash fit, hold the lashes up to your eyelid, by the fringe and keeping them away from the tear duct; smooth them (without glue) over your relaxed eye toward the outer corner. Mark the spot, take the lashes off the eye, and trim the outer end of the band so the lashes will stop where your own natural lashes do. Save the extra lashes for bottom fringe on your lower lids.

Now press the trimmed lash strip around your thumb to "press in" a curve. If your own lashes are straight, put in a soft curve with an eyelash curler. Apply a single coat of mascara to each of your own lashes to individually coat them.

Holding the lash strip in a crescent-moon curve, brush adhesive onto the ends of the last band with a toothpick. Press the last band to your eyelid, starting from the inner (tear duct) corner and following it to the outer corner. Use a clean toothpick to press it close to your own eyelashes. Hold both corners down for a few seconds to allow glue to dry snugly against the eyelid.

To remove, apply eye oil to the eyelid, wait a moment, lift the outer edge of the base strip and peel the lashes from the outer corner inward. Condition eyelid with eye oil. Set the eyelashes back in the box after cleaning and removing adhesive, according to the instructions in the kit.

Individual lashes: Individual lashes can be used only once, but can look so soft, if done well, that they can hardly be detected.

Purchase varied-colored-band type lashes in the color of your own lashes. With the fringe away from you, trim every third one just as you do for the strip application.

Next curl your own unmascaraed lashes with a hand lash-curler.

Now cut the strip into 3 to 5 sections. Holding one section with tweezers, dab the surgical glue (using the end of a toothpick or straight pin) onto the tiny strip at the base of the lashes, and spread it evenly.

Now act quickly, before the glue dries! Place the section along the lash line, thus thickening your own lashes (start with short lashes toward the nose, and work out the longer ones). The eye is relaxed. Use fingers or tweezers, whichever is most comfortable, but be careful not to bend the lashes. A hand mirror is easiest to use.

Continue the process, working your way to the outer corner of the lid and using the longer lashes where your lashes are longer. You may also apply several to the lower lid, shortened to match your natural ones.

Whether you're using the bands or the individual lashes, when the glue has dried (3-5 minutes), apply several light coats of mascara to both top and bottom lashes. Powder lashes before the final coat of mascara, and don't miss powdering the top of the upper lashes before mascaraing them, too.

To remove the artificial lashes, use your mascara removal technique. Then peel the lashes off from the base strips, if there's enough of the strip to catch hold of with fingers or tweezers. If not, rinsing will make the glue gummy and moist; the water and/or cleansing oil should loosen the lashes enough to come off. Discard the individual lashes.

Glamour Model Face Tool Checklist

Cosmetic Products

- ☐ Under-base tint, or pre-makeup
- ☐ Light concealer (and possibly medium-color too)
- ☐ Foundation/Makeup Base:
    - —lightest possible color
    - —ivory or beige family preferred
- ☐ Highlighter (shimmer or iridescent)
- ☐ Light Translucent Powder (and/or pearly loose powder)
- ☐ Eyebrow Powder
    - —light color
    - —dry cake brush-on powder
- ☐ Eye shadow
    - —vivid or dark colors, optional shimmer
- ☐ Eyeliner
    - —crayon, eyebrow pencil or powder, cake, or liquid
- ☐ Mascara (artificial lashes optional)
- ☐ Powder Blusher
    - —lots of shimmer (even metallic lights)
- ☐ Lipliner
    - —vivid colors
- ☐ Lipstick
    - —vivid colors
    - —frosted (or opaque)
- ☐ Lip Gloss (high sheen)

Cosmetic Tools

- ☐ Makeup "silk" sponge
- ☐ Powder complexion brush and powder pad
- ☐ Natural sea sponge
- ☐ Eyebrow brush
- ☐ Lipstick brush
- ☐ Mascara comb and eye shadow brush

Model Face—Glamour Formula

Complexion, Eyes, Lips

1. Glamour Complexion

Smooth on the under-base tint thinly, with sponge, to level and color-correct.

Dab concealer generously onto under-eye circles, shadows, blemishes, discolorations, flaws.

Contour with any other light creme products you want to use to sculpt or correct the face via lights and shadows.

Take a look in the Contouring chapter for more detail.

Lightly spread your foundation with a makeup sponge, avoiding eye area and the lips unless contouring. The correct color will need little blending to hairline.

2. Complexion Face Finishing

Pour loose translucent powder into the powder pad; fold the pad in half, with the powder on the inside. Then rub the two sides of the pad together so that the powder is ground into the pad and isn't loose on top of it. Lightly pat the face with the pad.

Dust some pearlized powder with a complexion brush, over the face, paying special attention to the bones, the entire eye circle, and the jawline. Rub in or brush off any excess.

Dampen a natural sea sponge, wring it "dry" in a towel, and lightly pat it over any dry areas, to "set" the makeup to last and look naturally perfect.

3. Glamour Contouring with Light Colors

Use any creme, pencil, or powder contour products that highlight—matte or frosted.

Eye Area: On top of your moisturizer you may use a very sheer, creamy, moist highlighter on the crowsfeet and fine lines at the outer corner of the eyes to help soften the lines visually. Often—with time and nourishing products—these lines may soften permanently.

Try this easy "olive-fork" method of highlighting the brow, outer-eye area, and upper cheekbone area with highlighter to emphasize your eyes.

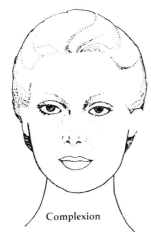

Complexion

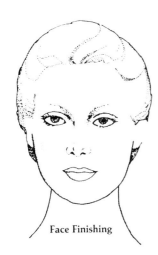

Face Finishing

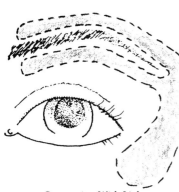

Contouring With Lights

The
Glamour
Face

Another highlight: With your white pencil or highlighter powder, draw a thin line the full length of the brow, just underneath it. (If you used pencil, you may now repeat, on top of the line, with highlighter powder, to set and enhance, if you like.) With the powder, you may also line the brow, above the brow from the highest point of the arch out toward the temple.

To further contour, you may brush the highlighter powder to travel parallel above your creme rouge on the cheekbone—the length of the cheekbone, to the temple. Also dust your jawline to "square" it for this image, if needed. Blur the contour "edges" lightly with makeup sponge.

4. Glamour Cheekbones

Barely dust the outer cheekbone ridge and hollow below it with your shimmery or iridescent powder blusher. Direct it from near the hairline down to, and in line with, the outer corner of colored iris of the eye.

Be careful not to overdo sculpting out the cheekbone hollows or making the front of your face rosy. This detracts from the eyes and lips of the Glamour formula, looking over-madeup and not true to its "image."

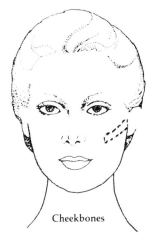

Cheekbones

5. Glamour Eyebrows

Lightly color or brush the brows into the "winged" brow shape.

Use this arch guide for the correct shape from the tear duct to the highest point of the arch. (If you've already shaped for Classic, you've got it.) Gently taper the outer half of the brow from the high point, to the outer corner, toward the hairline.

An alternative Glamour shape is the rounded eyebrow.

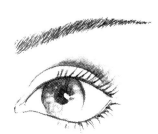

Winged Brow

6. Glamour Eyes

Artificial Eyelashes. If you use artificial lashes, here's the time to add the type of your choice. Whether you use false lashes or just stick to mascara, keep in mind that with a rounded Glamour eyebrow and/or for a round, starry-eyed Glamour eye, a few individual false lashes (or extra mascara) in the center of the lower eyelid are great.

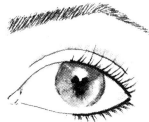

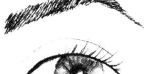

Soft Glamour Eyeliner

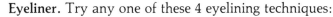

Eyeliner. Try any one of these 4 eyelining techniques:

Line upper and lower eyelids, as close to the skin just under the lashes as you can get. Even dot the eyeliner onto the skin between the lower lashes, if they're sparse. Then blur and smudge the lines to look smoky rather than drawn-on, giving the look of thicker lashes.

Use eyebrow or eyeliner powder, or pencil, crayon, or liquid eyeliner.

For soft Glamour, or to open up the eye, keep the eyeliner on the outer half of both the top and bottom lids, using pencil, powder, or soft crayon. Then blur and smudge the lines to look smoky rather than drawn on, giving the look of thick lashes.

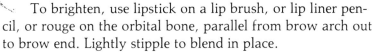

For mysterious Glamour, or to close up the eyes, line both eyelids from tear duct to outer corner. Then line the inside of the lower eyelids (between lashes and eyeball) with dark pencil.

Mysterious Glamour Eyeliner

To add size or drama, doming enhances the shape of the eye. Using your liner, begin with a thin line that gradually widens, or domes, over the center of the eyelid, and then tapers back down to a thinner line on the outer third of the eye.

To brighten, use lipstick on a lip brush, or lip liner pencil, or rouge on the orbital bone, parallel from brow arch out to brow end. Lightly stipple to blend in place.

Eye shadow. Choose from one of these techniques or use any one of your own:

Vertical eye shadow dramatizer.

Horizontal (crease) eye shadow dramatizer.

Horizontal (eyelid) eye shadow dramatizer.

Domed Eyeliner

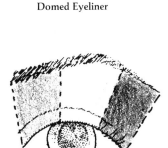

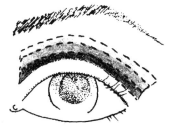

Vertical Eye Shadow Dramatizer

Horizontal (Crease) Eye Shadow

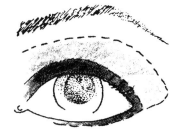

Horizontal (Eyelid) Eye Shadow

Mascara. Add several coats. Powdering before the last coat adds a lot more thickness, drama, and staying power.

7. Glamour Lips

Outline lips with vivid-color lip pencil, light or dark. You may exaggerate lips by drawing the liner just barely outside the lip line, or directly onto the lip line edge itself.

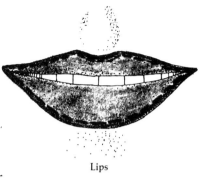

Lips

Add vivid lipstick, especially lightest or darkest colors, or frosted ones. Using a lip brush will allow a heavier concentration of the lipstick, and give it a smoother look as the lip cracks are filled. This technique also lasts longer than "tubed"-on lipstick.

You may apply the lipstick to just inside the lipliner, for a full-lip look, or over it to the outer edges. You may use a light, frost color inside and a darker color on the outer limits for an even fuller, more "kissable" look.

Touch on a coat of heavy gloss or colored slicker for added pizazz. (If it's a lipstick tube-type gloss, use your lipstick brush to apply the gloss before your lipstick!)

8. Glamour Wrap-Up

With a last swirl of the powder brush, add just the tiniest extra bit of pearlized powder to your cheekbones. Spray your hair into place if you wish. And turn back to the Check-Out, which appears earlier in this chapter, before you look into the mirror for that final glance to be sure you've got the Glamour formula.

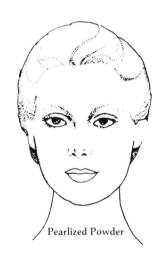

Pearlized Powder

Who is that stunning creature sparkling back at you? Why, it's you, in your most vivid, Glamour face, of course!

Chapter 5

Candlelight Basics

After 5:00 for Every Image

Rather than merely adding more makeup than you wear during the day, you want to capture every refraction of evening's lights as skillfully as you can. And you want to avoid turning muddy-looking, or fading into the foliage, in quirksome night-time light!

Looking your most sparkling is easy when you borrow some time-honored secrets long used in theatrical circles! These are the minor adjustments to make to your daytime face for evening's light. They're easy, quick, and you may already have the needed cosmetics.

1. Make your skin glow underneath your makeup.
2. Make your colors glow by using pink on evening "touch-points."
3. Make your eyes glow by using charcoal and white skillfully, while still being faithful to the formula for the face you're wearing: Classic, Earthy, Romantic, or Glamour.
4. Shimmer, Shimmer, Shimmer!

1. Candlelight Adjustment

Skin glow can be as fast as your speediest facial scrub. Strip down those dead cells, that oil and old makeup, to your squeaky-clean skin. You'll have a fresh glow that, by the way, helps your makeup go on more smoothly as well as revitalizing you for the evening ahead.

Obviously there's no substitute for the above; but if you are in a situation where you must go directly from your day into your evening, here are a few tips for making the transition as gracefully as possible.

If you're an oily skin, pass a cotton ball soaked with astringent, pH-balancer, or cool water over your face. If you can't manage that, blot your face with a tissue (don't rub!) to lift off any excess oil. Next lightly powder; even if you can't make your skin glow with a facial scrub, you can make it appear velvety with translucent powder. If you're a dry skin, smooth on just a little moisturizer after the astringent.

Now apply your cosmetics. Suit them to the image of your choice for the evening, and tailor that image to the rules of evening lighting.

2. Candlelight Adjustment

Color. Evening light drains away your color, washing out even the darkest brunette's features. In the evening, pink is for every face, regardless of natural coloring. The cooler the pink (more blue than yellow), the more flattering your "flush" will appear in evening lights. So pick the coolest one you're comfortable with. It can be bright—if that suits the image you've selected.

Your evening touch-points are temples, cheekbones, collar-bone hollows, earlobes, orbital bone (above eye crease, and below brow), earlobes, and cleavage (especially if you have some).

Cool pink should be dabbed on these points in a mixture of moisturizer and pink creme color.

3. Candlelight Adjustment

Charcoal and White. Isn't everything more one-dimensional looking at night? Don't trees look like cardboard when your car headlights pick them out? To avoid flat features, "pick them out" with charcoal-based colors for brow and eye makeup.

White also adds dimension especially in conjunction with the dramatic charcoals. White may be a highlighter (your coolest one for evening, please), or it may be the iridescent shimmer of your pearlized powder on temples, cheekbones, entire eye area, collar bones, and shoulders.

The white may also be your white pencil lining the inner eyelids (between lashes and eyeball). That trick certainly perks up tired "whites" and intensifies your eye color for evening light. Line along the underside of the entire length of the brows, too, for extra sculpting and dimension.

4. Candlelight Adjustment

Above all, shimmer, shimmer, shimmer. Starlight, moonlight, dim light, candlelight: they all were made for iridescent, shimmery, even metallic cosmetics, clothes, and accessories. Such lights flicker over your sparkle, making you look even prettier than in daylight! That pearlized powder is pure joy, especially when you're wearing either Romantic or Classic Face, which exclude metallic eye shadows, blushers, etc., in their formulas.

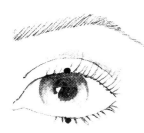

Iris Dots

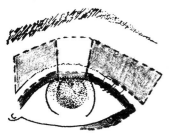

Vertical Eye Shadows

Extra secrets

5. Iris Dots. These little dots work wonders in making eyes larger in night-light. They are used by all but the Classic Face. With an iridescent, light-colored liquid eye shadow stick, place a dot on the top and lower eyelids. Place it directly in the center of each, on lid skin close to lashes. It will look a little obvious in your bathroom light; out it won't.

6. Vertical Eye Shadows. Long eyeliner and crease shadows are great for Earthy or Glamour eyes. Keep the center of the eyes shiny and light, though.

7. Eye Brighteners. Splashing cold water—or pressing a cold washcloth or cotton ball—onto your eyelids can reduce redness. So can eye drops, and Vitamin B6 if you think of it early! A quick nap, if you have time, reduces redness and brightens your eyes.

For a quick eye-area clean-up, lightly dip a cotton swab in moisturizer, and gently wipe your under-eyes to lift dark makeup that's crept down during the day. Follow with light powder, to prevent eye makeup from being attracted back down by the moisturizer.

8. Dual Lipliner. (For all except Romantic Face) Keep your lightest lipliner color on the outside, and your darkest color on the inside of the lip edges. (For instance, use white pencil outside lip edges, and red pencil on or inside lip edges.) Then add lipstick and gloss if your face is Glamour or Classic. Earthy gets just the gloss.

9. "3-D" Shadow. Add final eye shadow dust to Glamour or Earthy eyelids with charcoal color, sheer enough not to diminish sheen or darken color more than you like.

10. Spirit Revitalizer. If you have time, put your feet up and take a cat nap. Or soak your feet in a warm, fragrant tub, (or better yet, soak your entire self). Don't drink hot drinks or run the water blisteringly hot, unless you want to be slow-moving tonight: heat is enervating. If you need to be perky, finish your bath with an exhilarating rinse in almost-cold water.

One last luxury tip. While you're elevating feet, catnapping, or soaking in a warm bath tub, you can be using that time to revitalize your complexion as well.

3→20 Minute Miracle
Candlelight Skin Revitalizer

1. Thoroughly cleanse your face and throat, including a facial scrub if you like.
2. Generously apply a very fine eye or throat reconditioning oil to your entire face and throat; let it soak in for a moment or two.
3. On top of the oil, smooth on a clay-mineral masque, adding minute quantities of water only if absolutely necessary to get it to spread (the oil already on the skin should help).
4. Add a jot more oil to the outer corners of the eyes, or around the eyes, to extra-condition those areas while the masque is working on the rest of the face.
5. 3 to 20 minutes of resting with this masque should make you smoother and more glowing, make your makeup application much more successful, and add a new lift to your spirits. (Gentle oils and masques, with the longer resting time, produce the best results.)
6. Now rinse with warm water, and use a splash of cool to close pores and refresh eyes. Wipe a cottonball over your dried face to spread a bit of astringent, pH-balancer, or fragrant toner.
7. Proceed with your moisturizer and makeup—refreshed and ready for the evening as never before!

Chapter 6

Tips for Special Circumstances

Colorful Confessions

Your Altered Hair Color in the 4 Images and Color Keys

If your hair and general coloring benefit from altering your hair color, this section is for you. Take it with you to the beauty salon to assist your colorist there, or take it when you shop if you're a do-it-yourself colorist. A more detailed chart is provided at the end of this section for color students.

Color

Results of some hair products can augment your natural coloring or heighten your Image impact. For example, L'Oreal hair color products are predominantly muted shades, so if you prefer muted tones, you'll be likely to find just the right color in their line, especially if you know that you are *"Autumn/Muted/Sunset"* or *"Summer/Gentle/Sunlight."*

Clairol and Roux products, by contrast are predominantly clear tones, and whether you're looking for cool or warm clear colors, you can expect to find something you will like *("Winter/Contrast/Sunrise,"* and *"Spring/Light-Bright/Sunlight"*).

Henna products are best if you look good with muted or ashy hair coloring—often with a bronze cast. A tremendous color selection is available to the warm, muted coloring *("Autumn/Muted/Sunset").*

Frosting is best on those with cool, muted coloring *("Summer/Gentle/Sunlight")*. "Sun-In"—type streaking products are generally muted and warm *("Autumn/Muted/Sunset")*.

Image

To heighten your Image impact, remember that Classic and Romantic Images require closest-to-your-own-natural-hair-color look. Your choice for Classic can be a little sharper than for soft-focus Romantic, but remember that Classic, above all Images, needs to look shiny and healthy.

Predominantly one-color hair, rather than 3-D, is best for both Classic and Romantic Images.

Earthy colors and sunny streaks can add warmth to your down-to-earth look. Daylight should pick out natural highlights in your Earthy hair, so be sure to ever-so-subtly luminize, hair-paint, or sun-streak. If you look good in gentle reddish highlights, bring them out for Earthy or Romantic Face. Heavy metallic, bronze hennas, vivid colors, and obviously man-influenced hair colors spell Glamour.

Color your hair dramatically for one-color looks. If heavy frosting becomes you, Glamour Image is the place for it.

A Few Special Notes about Coloring.

Glamour hair colors are beautiful with a metallic shine. The cool, muted color key *("Summer/Gentle/Sunlight")* is the best key to wear frost. The warm, muted key *("Autumn/Muted/Sunset")* is the best key to wear henna.

The warm, clear key *("Spring/Light-Bright/Sunlight")* must be careful with blonding. Blonding products have a tendency to turn greenish and ashy, (the warm, muted key of *"Autumn/Muted/Sunset"*), especially if the hair is "mouse brown," ashy, or taupey to start with.

Hair Coloring Suggestions by Natural Coloring and by Image

Cool, clear	Warm, clear	Cool, muted	Warm, muted

Classic shiny with health, subtle, understated, medium shades, close to your own natural color

Cool, clear	Warm, clear	Cool, muted	Warm, muted
Dark brown, Brown-black, Silver, Flaxen blonde	Clear yellow, Clear amber, Medium brown, Solid color	Medium brown, Ash brown, Hair painting, One color, Luminize	Medium brown, Taupe auburn, Dark ash, One color

Earthy natural, sunny, sun-streaked, blonde or reddish tones, not too shiny

Cool, clear	Warm, clear	Cool, muted	Warm, muted
Brunette— medium brown to black, Luminize	Red, Straw, Honey brown, Strawberry-blonde, Luminize Lemon chamomile rinse, Non-white (yellow) hair painting	Mocha, Strawberry, Ash brown, Streaked blonde, Hair painting, Light frost	Yellow-gold, Brown, Red, Strawberry, Bronzy blonde, Golden, Sun-In Sun streaked

Romantic soft colors, best without streaks

Cool, clear	Warm, clear	Cool, muted	Warm, muted
Flaxen blonde, Brunette— brown and black, Strawberry, Luminize	Flaxen blonde, Medium brunette— brown, honey, amber, chestnut Red-black, Luminize	Mahogany, Medium brown, Natural blonde, Rosy brown, Pale cornsilk blonde, Luminize	Chestnut, Medium brown, Medium taupe, Honey brown, Pale Luminize

Glamour very dark, very light, vivid, brilliant, or metallic sheen

Cool, clear	Warm, clear	Cool, muted	Warm, muted
Dramatic ash, silver, or platinum blonde Auburn, Raven, blue-black, Snow-white, Cherry, Plum, Color crayons	Dramatic light red-gold, Darkest chestnut Red-black	Dark ash brown, Medium and deep brunette, Medium to heavy frost Ash blonde	Dramatic carrot or fiery red, Deepest taupe, Darkest Luminize

Men Will Make Passes at Lasses in Glasses

Eyeglasses for the 4 Images and Color Keys

One of the most exciting fashion statements around is greatly undervalued: eyeglasses! Eyewear can stylishly accessorize your beautiful Image. Or glasses can "make or break" your chosen image by augmenting or competing with everything else you've done to set your mood. Best of all, they can replace the need for eye makeup. When you're really in a hurry, just add this cachet-catcher, and you'll step out of a magazine.

If you wear glasses daily, it would be worth it to have at least two or three pairs—one for each of your favorite Images. After all, if you've pulled together everything from fragrance to hairstyle to state an image, why not use eyeglasses to promote your mood too?

The feelings of the Classic, Earthy, Romantic, and Glamour Images are all captured by today's beautiful eyeglasses. First determine the frame shape that best suits your face shape. Then determine colors and materials to suit your coloring, and whether the style suits your Image(s).

Choosing the Best Frame for Your Face Shape

If you're not sure which facial shape you have, look in the Contouring Primer and determine whether yours is a triangle, round, rectangle, diamond, square, or oval facial shape.

Your eyeglass frames should complement your face, repeating shapes you like, discouraging lines you don't. If your face is round, for example, and you like the look, you can wear a rounded frame, but if it's too round for comfort, try a frame that creates another line, maybe a horizontal bar or oblong to break the circle in half.

Small noses look best when the bridge of the glasses is rounded, slim, or high. Long noses can be "cut" by choosing a frame with a thick, low-slung, or straight bridge.

Glasses designed with upward curves or lines tend to lift the face, diminishing the sagging effects of aging.

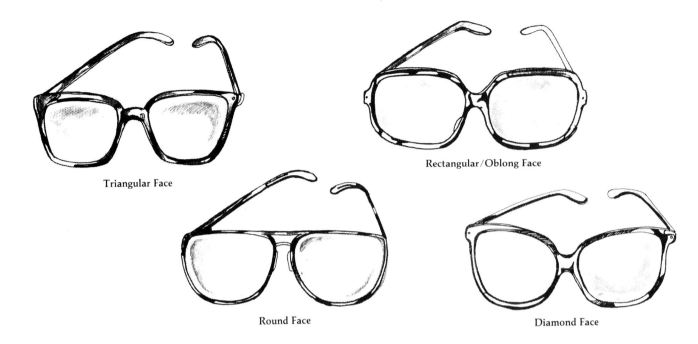

Triangular Face

Rectangular/Oblong Face

Round Face

Diamond Face

Triangular Faces

Choose frames that add width to the narrow end of the triangle. If your face shape is the standard triangle, frames with height at the top outside corners of the frame balance the face.

Round Faces

Choose non-rounded, horizontal shapes. Examples are: slender oblongs, square rectangles, and straight lines across the bridge of the nose.

Rectangular/Oblong Face

Choose frames with rounded edges that do not repeat the long, oblong shape. Frames that emphasize the horizontal rather than the vertical soften the long face—wider rather than taller. They extend past the temples.

Diamond Faces

Choose frames that create vertical, parallel lines at the upper sides of the face. These lines should break up that wideness when situated just inside the outline of that widest point.

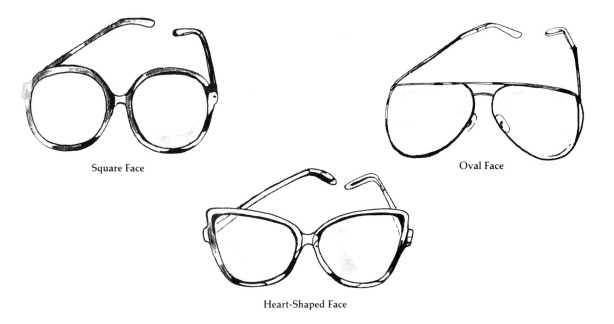

Square Face

Oval Face

Heart-Shaped Face

Square

Repeat the squares for an aggressively angular look. If you prefer, use rounded frames to reduce the angular squareness of the face.

Heart-Shape

To emphasize the heart-shaped face, choose slightly bowed or bow-shaped frames that are smaller and constricted in the center; both top and bottom edges should fan out and away from the face.

To minimize the heart-shape, choose a frame that flares away and down and is wider at the bottom frame edge than the top.

Oval Face

Virtually any frames that you like are flattering, so choose the colors, materials, shapes, and styles that flatter your individual facial features and the Images you prefer to wear.

Choosing Style, Material, and Color

Very small frames—that is, small in proportion to your face—project an Earthy Image, as do "aviator" glasses of all types. Frames in proportion to the face—where the amounts of glass above and below the eye are nearly equal—project the moderation of the Classic Image or the softer look of the Romantic Face. Oversize, dramatically designed frames always say Glamour.

The materials of the frames can also encourage your mood. Metal frames and tinted lenses can add to your Earthy aura. Old fashioned wire "specs" project "down-to-earth." Tortoise-shell or horned rims on squared or mildly rounded shapes spell Classic.

Lightly-colored, pastel, clear, milky, or barely frosty rims are often Romantic. Nothing too dramatic—just soft, lovely, and feminine. Some metal frames are even Romantic. They're not easy to find—look for medium-size and an indeterminate shape that is neither aviator nor small and John Lennon-looking.

For your Glamour Face, anything exaggerated goes if the color and shape suit you. Rose-colored lenses? Rhinestone-studded frames? Your glamorous look can range from classy designer trends to the latest bizarre innovations. Wrap-arounds are usually glamorous accessories, as are initials and monogram. When the upper half of the frame angles out and upward, you usually have a Glamour frame.

Half-glasses are flexible—they can go with any image in the right packaging. Very thin metal half-glasses with a Romantic Face and hairstyle can look romantic. Slightly heavier metal half-frames can look earthy with Earthy Face and hair that is straighter, even ragged—long or short. Tortoise-shell or businesslike dark and opaque half-frames look Classic with that Face and tidy hair. Exaggerated plastic frames—even adorned with such things as rhinestones and neck-chains—can be Glamour when worn with that Face and a severe hairstyle.

Color students—don't forget silver trims and frames are for cool coloring ("Winter/Contrast/Sunrise" and Summer/Gentle/Sunlight"). Gold is for clear, warm coloring ("Spring/Light-Bright/Sunlight"), and gold, coppery, or bronzy metals are for muted, warm coloring ("Autumn/Muted/Sunset").

Choose frame colors that harmonize with your natural coloring to enhance your coloring as well as your image.

You Ought to be in Pictures!

Putting Your Best Images in Front of the Camera

So you've got to be camera-ready? Whether for photograph or video film, these hints will help you make the most of photogenic self.

Black-and-White Photography

Black-and-white photography remains one of the best ways to achieve a becoming photograph. The camera smooths out awkward lines and can add angles you wish you really had!

You cannot wear too much makeup for this medium. The camera can absorb as much as you can pack, and you'll still look like you! With black-and-white, you needn't worry that your makeup colors might look garish. And makeup lines and angles are softened at the same time yours are emphasized.

Wear white and black clothing, if you like a crisp look, and use white and black cosmetics like highlighters, eyeliners, and mascara with a dramatic flourish. They look wonderful. Sparingly applied false eyelashes (especially the individual ones) look natural; heavily but well-applied false lashes look slightly artificial and beautifully dramatic.

Use plenty of contour powder on the outer cheekbones, the underside of the jaw, and anywhere else you'd like to thin, hollow, or sculpt. Use plenty of translucent powder to keep down the shine and add a velvety finish to your skin.

Tone down prominent eyelids with dark colors and highlight deep-set eyes with lights. Check through the contouring chapter for any special ideas. Black-and-white photography captures drama, so don't worry about color-keying your clothes or makeup. Use strong lines and intense colors, and you'll love the finished product.

Back-lit hair adds pizazz to any black-and-white photograph. This technique also helps "thicken" fine and thin hair.

Whether you're being photographed for color or black-and-white, examine past photos of yourself. Pick out the things you don't like about your hair, face, and clothes. Use your color, and makeup contouring, information to make improvements; add your Image techniques, and watch for the camera to find you lovely and stylish!

Color Photography

Whether you're just posing for a color still, or for video, film, or television, the techniques you want to employ for color photography differ from black-and-white.

Choose your most clear, brightly colored garments for the crispest picture. Never wear solid black or white garments. (Your palest blue will appear white!)

You can successfully wear unlimited concealer makeup, under-base tint, foundation, and powder, but keep the use of bright colors on your face to a minimum. Cheek color can look particularly glaring and overdone, and eyeliner overly dramatic.

When applying your makeup, remember that color film adds too much shine and drama to the skin. Use plenty of translucent powder and, if you like, apply it in the manner suggested for the Model Face in the Classic chapter.

Smudge eyeliner well to eliminate overly sharp lines around the eye. Keep artificial lashes as natural-looking as possible (usually this means individual rather than band lashes). Use flesh and cream tones to highlight wherever possible; iridescent, bright white looks very "hard" in color shooting, even if it looks great on you in person. Warm your dark contouring with a little flushed color if it looks too muddy to the naked eye; the camera would only make it muddier if you neglected to warm it up.

Lots of lip gloss and lights...camera...action!

Chapter 7

Skin Care Basics

Preparing the Artist's Canvas

So much has been written about basic skin care that it's a marvel that everyone isn't enjoying beautiful, healthy skin. Perhaps women (and men) still don't think of their skin as the largest organ of the body, which needs cleansing, rest, exercise, nutrition, and protection just as do their other major organs.

Beautiful skin is a mirror of your health and way of life. Seven easy steps toward a glowing complexion are:

1. Cleanse
2. Exfoliation/Stimulation
3. Skin Tightening/Stimulation
4. Restore pH Balance (acid mantle)
5. Moisturize
6. Nourish
7. Protect

Today's modern products now help you take each of these steps quickly and effectively. Before taking any steps, however, you need to know your skin type. Then you'll be able to make well-educated choices of products and care.

If you haven't indexed your skin lately, try the following Skin Test to determine your current type of complexion.

Then review the seven easy skin-care steps, and take a peek at "A Dozen 'Did You Know That?' Basics," and a few modern-lifestyle tips.

Skin Test

Read each question, and check off the statements that sound most like your skin. The column with the most checks indicates your skin type.

1. Even without moisturizer, my makeup base:

☐ looks oily and shiny quickly
☐ can cake and look splotchy
☐ becomes darker or orange in color

☐ shines on my nose, chin, and forehead (the rest of my makeup looks all right)

☐ does not glide on easily
☐ lacks luster and gleam
☐ looks dry 2-3 hours later

☐ pulls instead of glides when I apply it
☐ looks dry and crepey within 2-3 hours of application
☐ much powder makes my face look dry

2. If I use soap and water to clean my face:

☐ it feels fresh and clean

☐ my nose and chin feel fresh, but my eyes and cheeks feel tight and dry

☐ my skin feels drawn and dry
☐ usually I need to moisturize

☐ it gets positively tight, flaky, and dry
☐ it may look blotched, red, or irritated
☐ I must immediately moisturize
☐ my face soaks up moisturizer

3. If I use cleansing cream to clean my face:

☐ I don't feel clean
☐ I feel greasy
☐ my pores get clogged

☐ I seem to have a film on my face
☐ my nose area feels greasy

☐ my face feels clean
☐ but not "squeaky" clean
☐ my face feels softened

☐ my face feels clean
☐ it helps soften any patchy areas
☐ my face feels nice and soft

4. My skin naturally:

- [ ] tends toward clogged, large pores
- [ ] gets oil "slicks" in nose and chin area
- [ ] tends to produce blackheads, whiteheads. and blemishes
- [ ] I suntan easily and seldom burn

- [ ] has average pores
- [ ] has larger pores in nose and chin area
- [ ] may produce some blackheads, whiteheads, and blemishes

- [ ] has basically unnoticeable pores
- [ ] may be dry in winter or after sunbath
- [ ] eye wrinkles may be forming

- [ ] is thin and sensitive
- [ ] may look a bit red or rough
- [ ] may feel a bit rough
- [ ] gets dry in patches and sometimes flakes
- [ ] is forming or has formed fine or heavy lines and wrinkles early
- [ ] sunburns easily

My skin type is:

| Oily | Oily to Normal | Normal to Slightly Dry | Dry to Extremely Dry |

Daily Cleansing

Before we discuss your face cleansing regimen, let's take a look at a First Rule of Skin Care: **Always use lukewarm water on your skin.**

Why? On a regular basis, using extremes of temperature—either very hot or cold—can be harmful to your skin.

Very hot water, for example, dramatically opens up the pores and brings sub-cutaneous oils to the surface. This has often been suggested as a way of cleansing the skin, but it is very harsh. Years of repeating this action can increase oiliness, and enlarge pores by permanently stretching out their elasticity.

If you doubt the rough effect of cold temperatures, notice your own face during cold weather. Then go home and start turning on your skin's best friend: a tepid not cold tap!

If it's available and you can afford it, using either distilled or natural spring water is better for your skin's health. Those waters contain fewer harsh salts and industrial chemicals. Spring waters also have a high natural mineral content.

And as long as you've invested in this smart water, you'll benefit from drinking it, too! The complexion responds beautifully to plenty of fluids, and they will be reflected in your moist, lustrous skin. Efficient elimination of toxins keeps your skin lovely; clean water is essential to this cleansing process.

If you've been using facial tissues, toilet tissue, or other paper products to "tissue" off your cleanser, you might be chagrined to look at those wood fibers under a microscope. Optometrists all over the country recommend avoiding use of paper products on eyeglasses because they scratch. Save your delicate complexion from the same fate—switch to sea sponges, real cotton, 100 percent cotton washcloths, of some other gentle method.

The value of the very best skin-care treatment is diminished greatly without good stimulation. Stimulation is so vital that many products that meet any of the seven skin needs also include ingredients to promote better circulation and stimulation.

In the end, exercise can promote a healthy blood supply like no external products can, and skin that is the recipient of regular stimulation through exercise will double, triple, or quadruple its beauty. Yes, it's boring to talk about the blood bringing food and oxygen to the skin, and carrying away garbage, but it is, after all, the happy result of all this water drinking, exercising, and cosmetic stimulation.

Cleanser Product Basics

Ideal cleansers penetrate layers of the skin and return dirt and oils to the skin's surface to be rinsed away. Unless your hormone balance is affected by medicine or age, you should not have a dramatically defined "T" zone: that extremely oily area through the forehead, nose, and chin. Modern cosmetics have made that problem obsolete by designing a wide range of cleansers for every possible skin type. A "T" zone usually indicates:

1. a change in hormone balance (can be caused by medicine, diet, lifestyle)
2. —or more commonly, use of products that are too harsh or strong for your skin.

Harsh products cause the oil production to increase in an attempt to off-set the loss of oils caused by the product.

What's Best for Daily Cleansing?

Today's environment offers a depressing variety of daily pollutants that are attracted like magnets to old makeup, naturally-accumulating skin secretions, and dead skin cells. We require a matching variety of cleansing products more than ever before.

All skin types respond to the balanced use of alternating products, so that your skin does not become immune to the benefits of one product used exclusively. Even in cleansing products, dry skins generally require additional moisturizing oils and humectants; oily skins require few.

Whatever you do, if your cleanser is designed to deodorize your armpits, keep it away from your face!

Cleanser products containing a high degree of naturally alkaline ingredients, soaps, or detergents tend to dry the skin and are designed—and best—for oilier skin types. Milky cleansers containing these ingredients usually penetrate to clean more deeply than soaps. There are even some liquid cleansing oils for the oily and large-pored skin that act like solvents on the skin.

Cleansing lotions are ideal for oily-to-normal skin types, and for normal-to-slightly dry. They are more water-soluble, having a higher water content, and still penetrate to lift dirt without really drying the skin.

Cleansing creams, a derivative of the "cold cream" family, contain ingredients other than the basic oils, waxes, and water of the cold-cream formulas, usually to provide additional services to the skin. Oily-to-normal skins prefer rinsing off these products, while normal-to-dry may wish to remove them only with their freshener/toner, or a (tepid!) damp washcloth.

Dry skins thrive under the application of moisturizing and liquifying cleansers, which contain a greater quantity of oils and waxes and a lesser quantity of water. Body heat warms these products, and they melt into the skin quickly upon contact. The effects are warm (as opposed to the cool feeling of cold creams), soothing, and softening. They leave the precious oil reservoirs of the skin intact. Some products may even leave behind the barest oil residue as a protective shield to keep natural moisture from leaching out of the skin.

Washing/bathing products—cream or lotion—are cleansers in their most water soluble forms. They are often ideal for the normal skin types. Bath oils are best for dry body skin.

Exfoliation/Stimulation

There has never been a better time to enjoy the sensations and benefits of deep pore, exfoliating skin-cleansing and stimulating. Instead of standing in the kitchen up to your neck in pots and blenders full of oatmeal, cucumbers, and fine cleansing grains, you can now head straight to your favorite cosmetic source for revitalizing treatments.

Pore congestion is part of our modern environment. Air pollution alone contains radiation, asbestos, sulfur, and hydrocarbons, to say nothing of water pollution. Add to that our makeup, and the natural skin secretions and dead surface skin cells that have always built up on the skin, and the total is clogged pores! Systematic decongestion of your pores with a deep-pore cleanser, which primarily sloughs off such build-up, is the way to remove that crust that's adding the look of years, not beauty, to your complexion.

Exfoliants are vital to strip away what you may have thought were your years creeping up on you! Many ideal exfoliant formulas support skin tissue and mildly stimulate circulation while they degrease, declog, and strip away. The new skin beneath is gleaming, soft, younger, and beautiful. Some "wrinkles" are merely cracks in this crust build-up; strip it away and find out what a hidden treasure you have under there! Regular use equals regular radiance.

What's Best for Deep-Pore Exfoliation?

All deep-pore exfoliants contain some granular substance that can produce a stripping-away action.

If you determined that your skin is currently oily, you'll want a scrub that features either greater or rougher grains, but be sure to choose one in a base that won't scratch your skin or destroy your natural skin ecology. If you strip too deeply, your oil glands respond by over-producing, just as with cleansers.

You're also baring defenseless skin to a hostile, bacteria-riddled world. Oily skins may use an exfoliant daily, and a damp sea sponge will perk up its action.

Dry-skin types need exfoliation too and will respond to the gentlest scrubbing with gentle products. Be sure the base of your product contains some ingredient—humectants, or natural properties (like those in honey, for example)—to buffer your sensitive skin and to ensure that your skin's moisture content is retained. Use only water and a gentle touch when applying exfoliants to a dry-skin type.

Oily-to-normal and normal-to-dry skin types thrive on a variety of applications. Try adding more water, or even throat oil, and gentle sea sponge scrubbing action if you're more dry than oily. All skin types should use a gentle, circular motion. Work up a real lather with less water and more sea sponge if you're more normal or oily.

And remember: whatever your skin type, be gentle.

Skin Tightening/Stimulation

Another method of deep-pore attention is the use of masques. Their primary purposes are:

1. tightening loose skin,
2. closing pores, and
3. increasing circulation.

As you can see, masques are very different from scrubs.

With age, weather, diet, and lifestyle, pores relax and lose their elasticity. They become larger and coarser-looking, and harder to keep clean. While you're stimulating your skin, you can be tightening these pores by adding a masque to your skin care kit. They supplement the cleansing process by drawing out impurities deeply imbedded in the skin. Contrary to popular belief, even dry skins benefit from an occasional skin-tightening treatment.

Daily Restoring of the pH-Balance (acid mantle)

Does this sound like a chore? It's actually one of the quickest and most pleasant steps of skin care: the use of refreshing toners, astringents, or fresheners that are acid-pH.

If you use a toner/freshener with cotton puffs, here's a pre-balancer basic: always use only real cotton on your face.

Many cosmetic "puffs," pads, and even face cloths now contain rayon and other man-made fibers that are very harsh to the skin. Try using real cotton to cleanse eye makeup from one eye, and a rayon cosmetic puff from the other eye. You can feel how much less the real cotton irritates the eye tissue. Use only 100 percent cotton: cloths, old cotton diapers, or cotton from pill bottles can be convenient.

Your skin has a delicate acid veil, called your acid mantle, that evenly covers every inch of your epidermis. This covering fights harmful bacteria and keeps your skin in perfect natural balance so that its cells can all work together. Fatigue, a diet high in refined sugars and other non-foods, pollutants, and alkaline products are among the factors that contribute to disturbing the skin's carefully supported coat of armor.

When you disturb it long enough and badly enough, it bites back, disturbing you with such reactions from its arsenal as rough, reddened skin, breaking out, fine lines, patchy areas, splotches, peeling, cracking, and "skin ache." Your skin stands up for itself; don't make an enemy of it!

In order to clean efficiently, you must disturb your acid mantle slightly (any time you wash it, this happens). When you immediately restore the mantle, there's no harm done. Good toners not only complete the cleansing process, they also restore this acid pH-balance.

What's Best for Restoring pH-Balance?
Always use a toner to complete your cleansing process—even for your easiest wash-and-wear-face. Your choice of product depends upon where your skin type fits on the oily-to-very-dry range.

Astringents are usually suggested for oily skins because of their "dehydration" capabilities, often based on witch hazel or alcohol or one of its derivatives. Careful—don't strip the skin of oil with a product that has a high percentage of alcohol, or with too-frequent astringent usage, or you'll have Texas-sized wells gushing to try to restore a little moisture to that parched skin!

Fresheners usually connote use by normal skins, and toners by the dry-to-very-dry. Toners usually have very little alcohol.

Moisturizing

You get thirsty during the day, and so does your skin! Moisturization does not necessarily mean oilization. As a matter of fact, oily skin caused by over-washing and harsh astringents responds to the addition of a light, mild humectant moisturizer like a thirsty person to a glass of water. You actually calm the oil gland activity down as the skin becomes less dehydrated.

Good moisturization is accomplished primarily by two compounds: oil and water.

Oily, creamy, or even greasy products can bring relief to dry skin. Oily substances coat the skin so that the skin's natural moisture doesn't evaporate as quickly. The point to understand here is that oil helps save moisture; it does not provide moisture. Water is water, and oil can never take its place, but it can and does help preserve your natural water resources.

Are you wondering if there are products that actually provide valuable moisture? Yes; "humectant" is a broad term for such agents, and many cosmetics use water itself as a prime ingredient.

So your moisturizing product will probably have both water and an oil-based ingredient. It should help "glue down" loose surface cells and scales, providing you with a smoother, softer look and feel (which helps the makeup go on more evenly and easily, too!) And it should act as a barrier to moisture loss by the skin by reducing evaporation of water from the skin. Skin cells with plenty of moisture will be elastic and supple.

Oily skin types don't always need moisturizer on a daily basis. They may get enough moisture and oil protection from their cleansers, toners, and makeup. Perhaps a dry area around the eye or throat could use a bit of beautifying oil at night or in sun or snow. Or perhaps an occasional dot of moisturizer is wanted for those times when rough weather or living set up a few dry patches on the face; moisturizers with very high water content and little wax are best.

Dry skins, which already lack water, should look not only to their moisturizers, but also to the climate, low humidity, cold wind, sun and even factors like exposure to soap and detergents, poor diet, and genetics to pin down causes of dry-skin problems before choosing or changing moisturizers. Your moisturizer needs may change if you make some lifestyle improvements. You may need several different kinds of moisturizers to change with the seasons.

(And remember the tip about rotating products so the skin doesn't become "immune.")

One fast water-restorer for temporarily dried skin is to pat the face with distilled water and then apply a generous coat of a very heavy nutritive oil. As the oil "melts" into the face, the dehydrated skin seems to absorb that water as well as the oil.

What's Best for Moisturizing?

More than any other skin care item, you'll have to try it to see if you like it. Knowing whether you need a greater or lesser oil content helps. Your primary goal is to find a product—or several products so you can rotate them according to the time of year, the time of the month, or the time of the day or evening—that will act as a primary water supply for your skin.

Moisturizer implies a medium-range product; emollient creams usually support skin that needs "heavier" (high oil content) lubrication against evaporation. Preparations for oily skins contain high levels of amino acids and water.

Nourishing Your Skin

Vitamins, minerals, protein compounds, and amino acids. Enzyme/nutrient-rich diet, and treatment creams and lotions. These are some of the many sources of nourishment available to your skin—inside and out. They can add a luster to your skin and give it a special glow. Nourishing the skin should be an inside-out process for your most vivid results!

Again, stimulation plays an active part. Whether you stand on your head, wear a masque, or jog around the block, getting the blood supply to the face increases the availability to the skin cells of nutrient-rich blood. And where does your blood get all of those nutrients? From your diet, of course!

If you are feeding your body foreign substances like cell-withering sodium chloride (either the processed table salt kind, or any kind in excess), wrinkling caffeine, wrinkling and spot-producing refined grains and sugars, or other non-foods, that's what you'll be bringing to your skin.

You are not only what you eat, but what you absorb! When your stress level is up, digestion of nutrients is down. Inhaling scalding, unchewed food on the run compounds the problem. Have you ever noticed how dull your skin gets under that kind of pressure? Circles and wrinkles show up more, and makeup doesn't go on smoothly?

Use the best of modern diet technology and bring along a thermos of protein drink from your blender, a container of yogurt, or even cheese, nuts, fruits, and vegetables when you know you won't have time for a meal. Take a few minutes, relax, and chew slowly. You'll be able to absorb those lovely life-giving substances from your food much better, and your skin and hair will reward you for it.

Topical nourishment is always an option. Dermatologists have been prescribing topical oils and creams for years, particularly those rich in fats and Vitamin A. Beware of mineral oil as either an inner or outer skin-nourishing treatment; it has no minerals or fats, and is a petroleum-based product that does not nourish your beauty or health.

Throat and eye emollients and specifically prepared night creams and oils are often rich in nourishing lubricants. They are too rich to be worn under makeup or with contact lenses, although if those details don't intrude on your day, you may like to wear such products while sunbathing, snow skiing, and during other outdoor exposure.

You will find products that are wonderful for your skin in the massive array of nutritive treatments and conditioning products available today.

What's Best in Nutrients?

Again, your needs dictate. Since none of these products can make miracle claims, you'll need to determine how you'd like to care for your skin first, and then look for ingredients that help achieve those results:

Vitamin A is often used for complexion and hair health, and for good resistance to infection.

Vitamin E is often used for skin elasticity and repair, as well as to soften and fight wrinkles.

Honey, used externally, helps regulate and maintain the skin's moisture content.

Some herbs have natural antiseptic, astringent, or circulation-stimulation properties—both internally and externally—and are power-houses of vitamins and minerals.

Proteins, enzymes, minerals, vitamins, collagen, RNA, elastin—there's a space-age collection of scientific discoveries out on the shelves for you to pick from to help you stay your loveliest!

Winning horse-trainers, dog-trainers, and every veterinarian will tell you that if you want to ensure that your animal has an especially beautiful coat, see that it gets rest, exercise, sunshine, and special oils and nutrients for sleek beauty.

Protection

Modern living has created a modern cosmetic need—that of skin protection from a harsh environment. As a result, many cosmetic companies have added some protection products to their lines, or ingredients to their products, to help barricade the skin from harmful particles and gases.

Talc is a particularly adept cosmetic defender, so look for makeup bases, foundations, and protection products containing this naturally repelling substance. "City skin" is no longer exclusive to metropolises like Pittsburgh, Los Angeles, and New York. Everyone gets their share of pollutants, so include exfoliation, pH-restoring, moisturizing and protecting in your skin care program.

8 "Did You Know That?" Skin-Care Basics

Did you know that:

1. Your "ring" or 4th finger is least muscularly developed and is the best finger to use when applying skin care treatments or blending makeup? Without great strength, it won't pull the not-very-elastic face tissue so roughly.

2. It's estimated that after 15 minutes or more of ultra-violet ray exposure, those rays begin damaging the skin? If you live in the sunbelt, you may want to use a PABA-based sunscreen and lip balm to help offset the skin/sun response.

3. The warmth of the sun's rays brings extra oils up to the skin's surface? This can enlarge pores over a length of time and may cause your skin to become oilier in the summer, making makeup darken or change color.

4. The moment you step out of a warm shower, while your pores are receptive, relaxed, and open, is the best time to apply nutrient-rich treatment oils and creams to the dry throat, face, and body? Also a good time to exfoliate and really clean out those pores.

5. When you're under the hairdryer, you need to protect delicate facial and eye tissue from damaging dehydration effects? Lubricate your face,

especially your eye/throat areas, with emollients or protective moisturizers.

6. You can use gravity to increase your beauty? Just always remember that it pulls down. Redirect blood to feed your face, and gravity to pull the other way for a few minutes, by using a slant board, or yoga positions, or lying down with your feet elevated and your head down. Let the blood rush to your face. And wear a bra to provide a resting shelf for some of that connecting tissue that's trying to sag!

7. Green plants in your bedroom will give you extra oxygen, purify your air, and help with humidity control while you sleep?

8. The hours of sleep before midnight seem to be the best for beauty sleep? Who knows why. But try sleeping from 9:30 p.m. to 6:30 a.m. and then from midnight to 9 a.m. the next day. If you're over 25, you'll see the difference in your face immediately. You may feel it, too. If you see the face difference, try taking catnaps if you're a real night owl and concerned about those sags and bags on your face.

When Prevention Is Better Than Cure

Smoking

If you're a smoker, have you seen the 1971 study by Dr. Harry W. Daniell, published in the *Annuals of Internal Medicine,* entitled "A Study in the Epidemiology of Crow's Feet"? We know that regardless of gender, there is a "striking" association between wrinkling and cigarette smoking.

Once you hit the 40 to 49 age bracket, you are likely to appear as wrinkled as a non-smoker 20 years older chronologically, according to the study. Nicotine restricts capillaries and blood vessels, reducing their capacity to bring nourishment and oxygen to your skin, especially the area around the eyes.

The Sun

Your skin is exposed to two kinds of ultra-violet rays when you expose it to the sun, and damage is believed to begin to occur after 15 minutes of exposure. Block those rays with sunscreen lotions, lip balms, and nose-cover products containing PABA or benzehenone. Protection rankings of 2 to 15 can be found on the label: 15 is the strongest, a sun block.

Improper Fad Diets

According to Dr. Peter M. Miller, author of *The Hilton Head Metabolism Diet*, metabolically your body's best fuel is a combination of nutrients in the following formula: 15 percent protein, 55 percent carbohydrate, and 30 percent fats.

On fad and crash diets that are unbalanced and deprive you of the best metabolic balance, you can become deficient in one or more of those nutrition elements, or disrupt the healthy ratio.

If you become deficient in carbohydrates you begin converting your body's proteins into carbohydrates and become protein-deficient. You're burning muscle instead of fat. Extended protein deficiencies show up in dull, thin hair; loose, sagging skin and muscle tone; and weak nails. Additionally, not eating a well-balanced diet means your skin is not getting the necessary full spectrum of vitamins, minerals, and enzymes.

The Pill

The chemical changes induced by birth control pills are similar to those that occur during pregnancy. According to Mead Johnson Laboratories, one manufacturer of the pill, 75 to 85 percent of women taking oral contraceptives may need as much as 25 mg. of Vitamin B6 daily as compared to the 1 to 2 mg. required by non-pregnant women not taking the pill, and the approximately 10 mg. requirement of pregnant women. Additionally, the pill seems to increase some women's need for Vitamin B-2, Vitamin C, Vitamin B-12, Zinc, and Folic Acid.

All of these nutrients affect your skin and hair beauty, for better or for worse, as well as your general health.

Use of the pill can cause "pregnancy mask," or "liver spots," a condition of heightened skin pigmentation which mottles the skin in patches. These spots can also occur with sun overexposure and with aging. Limit your ultraviolet exposure and increase your use of sun block products if you have a tendency toward these spots, or if you're on the pill and want to avoid them.

Many women have found that supplementing their food with B Vitamins and Folic Acid also diminishes this spotting.

Dermatologists have developed dermabrasion techniques to help. Sometimes regular use of an exfoliant scrub on the darkened patches that rise to the skin's surface can help fade them, if the new skin that grows beneath is normal. The effect is one of gradual diminishment.

A Contouring Primer

Contouring With Makeup to Visually Correct Flaws

Contouring your face with makeup is a creative and surprisingly easy way to beautify your face. Contouring can bring about the illusion of dramatic improvements to your face shape and individual features so that they conform to our current standard of beauty. Whether you do a little or a lot of contouring, don't forget to keep in mind the makeup guidelines of whichever Image you're wearing!

Contouring makes use of lights and shadows, and can be produced by many available makeup products. The techniques used here are designed to suit standard commercial cosmetics, rather than contour products created for theatrical makeup, professional makeup artists, or plastic-surgery patients. The techniques are simple and you probably have some of the cosmetics on hand. Your artist's tools are:

Lights (highlighting, light colors)—Bring forward. Lift out. Make narrow and sharply angular.

Shadows (darker, contour colors)—Recede. Sink back. Enlarge. Hollow.

Any cosmetic that you enjoy using and that is light or dark may be used to contour. For contouring with shadows, try foundation, rouge gels, and powder blushers all darker than your usual shade. For contouring with lights—highlighting—try light or pearlized translucent powder, a light-tone cover stick or creme, or a highlighter in any of these forms. Use light, translucent powder for highlighting.

Determine Your Face Shape

Step 1

Pull your hair completely away from your face. Look straight ahead into a mirror. With an eyebrow pencil, eye crayon, or lipstick, trace around the outer line of your reflected face onto the mirror, or, use a photograph of yourself looking straight at the camera with your hairline showing. Outline your face on tracing paper or draw on the photograph itself.

Step 2

Now, look at the shape you've drawn, and decide which of the seven face shapes it most closely matches. At first glance, it may look like more than one shape; take your time, decide which one it looks most like.

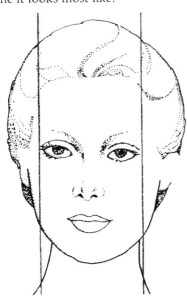

The seven face shapes:

- Triangular
- Round
- Rectangular/Oblong
- Diamond
- Square
- Heart (Upside-Down Triangle)
- Oval

If you're still not sure of your face shape, dissect the drawing of your face with a grid like the diagram left. Draw a vertical line down the length of the face on both sides, from the hairline above the forehead, in line with the outer corner of the eye, down to the jaw. The amount of face outside the two vertical lines helps you discover your facial shape.

Triangular. Is there very little of your face at the top, outside of the vertical lines you drew? And is there more at the middle, outside of the lines, and even more at the jawline outside? Your face shape is a triangle.

Round. Outside the vertical lines, is there more of the face near the ears, and gradually less curving upward and downward? And are "upward and downward" about equal? Your face shape is round.

Rectangular/Oblong. Is there very little to almost none, of your face outside of the vertical lines you drew? And is it the same width whether you look at the top, the middle, or the bottom sides of the face? Your face shape is a rectangle.

Diamond. Is there very little, to almost none, of your face outside of the vertical lines you drew? But what is outside is a little wider near the cheekbones and ears, and that same middle then angles sharply in, to be narrower above and below the middle? And are "above and below" about equal? Your face shape is a diamond.

Square. Is there a lot of your face outside the vertical lines you drew? And is it equal, from top to bottom? Your face shape is a square.

Heart (Upside-Down Triangle). Is there very little of your face, at the jawline, outside of the vertical lines you drew? And is there more at about the eye level, outside of the lines, and even more at forehead level, outside? Your face is heart-shaped.

Oval. Oval is considered by many to be the loveliest and most adaptable face shape. There is neither very little nor very much face outside the vertical lines you drew. And what is outside very gently curves from a hint wider at the eye/ear level, to slightly narrower at the forehead and jaw levels, which are almost equal to each other in width. Your face shape is oval.

Contour Your Face Shape

Now that you have diagnosed the shape of your face, your next step is to use contouring techniques to visually alter your face shape, emphasizing the shape if you like it, or downplaying it if you don't.

Triangular. To break up the triangle

- As much as you can—within the makeup guidelines of the Image you've chosen—place your rouge in broad, rectangular bands, from the hairline in toward the nose (no closer than the pupil of the eye). Stay high on the cheekbones.
- Highlight forehead and temples, to add width to the upper half of the face, if not covered with hair.
- When you want maximum correction, the triangle of features of Classic Face places a reverse shape-within-a-shape : an upside-down triangle. Earthy Face also adds fullness to the narrow upper face.
- Accessories and hairstyles are best when full at the top of the head, and broad across the forehead and even extended horizontally beyond. Hair should not be full at the jawline.
- Avoid ruffled necklines, which add fullness to the lower face. Closed-neck collars and necklines are best.

Round. You may wish the face to appear thinner. Also, since rounded faces tend to look girlish, you may wish to keep hair and makeup sophisticated. To thin the face:

- As much as you can—within the makeup guidelines of the Image you've chosen—place your rouge in triangles in the outer cheeks, with the highest point of the triangle rising toward the outer corner of the eye.
- Also use darker powder blusher to deeply sculpt out the hollows under the cheekbones within that triangle shape.
- The triangle of features of the Classic Face and the vertical lines of the Earthy reduce the round look. The one Image that looks wonderful emphasizing the round face is the Romantic Face even though you'll be using a round rouge shape instead of the contouring triangular rouge shape.

- Avoid severely short or sleeked-back hairstyles. To interrupt the roundness, use a definite side part and an asymmetrical hairstyle and avoid round or tiny accessories.
- Avoid rounded, scoop necklines. Use vertical clothing lines and v-neck lines to add angles to the roundness.

Rectangular/Oblong. To add width, as well as to shorten, the narrow, long face:

- As much you can—within the makeup guidelines of the Image you've chosen—place your rouge in somewhat narrow, horizontal bars, high on the cheekbones (not down near the cheek hollows, or across the face center toward the nose).
- To shorten the face a bit, use rouge—or darker foundation, powder, blusher, or other contouring products—to darken the chin.
- When you want maximum correction, choose an image that adds horizontal width to the center of the face: Earthy or Classic.
- Accessories and hairstyles should add width and fullness to the sides of the face around eyes, cheekbones, and ears.
- Avoid wearing long v-neck and vertical lines at the neckline. Use high necks, ruffles at the neck-line, and bateau (boat-neck) necklines to shorten the length of the face.

Diamond. To give a softer and fuller look to the sharp angles at top and bottom of the sides of the face:

- As much as you can—within the makeup guidelines of the Image you've chosen—place your rouge in rounded shapes, high on the cheekbones (not down near the cheek hollows, or across the face—center toward the nose). The more circular the rouge shape, the more flattering.
- When you want maximum correction, the rounded Romantic Image often softens the angles of the diamond/oblong face. Or the carefully sculpted brows and features of the triangle of the Classic Face can create a distracting shape-within-the-shape.
- Accessories and hairstyles should add fullness at the top of the head and below the ear, to widen the narrow angles.
- Avoid narrow v-neck lines, which can lengthen the face. Use high-necks and ruffles at the neckline to round out and shorten the face shape.

Square.

- As much as you can—within the makeup guidelines of the Image you've chosen—place your rouge in the shape illustrated: an almost-triangle, on its side. The "point" of the triangle of rouge should be in line with the pupil of the eye; the broad "base" of the triangle is to the outside of the face, toward the hairline and ears and not more than $\frac{1}{2}$ to 1-inch lower than the earlobes.
- Makeup that emphasizes the cheekbones softens the square. Darken the outer corners of the jaw to soften its lines and make them recede.
- To de-emphasize the angularity of the square face, choose Romantic Image. To suit its angularity, the Classic Image.
- Accessories and hairstyles that emphasize the cheekbones and the mid-line of the face are most flattering. Bangs and waves at the temple also soften the square.

- Avoid square necklines or large, square, boxy earrings if you have an aggressively square facial structure.

Heart-Shape. Since heart-shape is considered charmingly feminine, you may want to emphasize the shape. If you don't care for the shape, or just feel that your chin is too narrow or pointed, you may soften the shape. Whether you emphasize or de-emphasize the heart shape, the rouge application is the same:

- As much as you can—within the makeup guidelines of the Image you've chosen—place your rouge in broad, rectangular bands, from the hairline in toward the nose (no closer than the pupil of the eye). Stay high on the cheekbones.

To emphasize the heart-shape:

- Highlight forehead and temples (if not covered with hair) to add width to the upper half of the face. Long eyelashes and rosebud lips are best with the romantically presented heart-shaped face.

- Use darker, powder blusher to sculpt out the hollows under the cheekbones, down toward the lips.

- The Images that most strongly emphasize the heart shape are Classic and Earthy. Romantic Image best enhances the femininity of the heart-shaped face.

- Accessories and hairstyles are fuller at the top of the head than at the jawline. Upswept at the sides (such as with hair combs) and off the forehead (especially if you have a "widow's peak") further emphasize the feminine appeal. If you want bangs, wear them full, and curly if possible; be sure the hair at the jaw level is not full.

- Use v-neck and "sweetheart" necklines to repeat and emphasize the heart-shape.

To de-emphasize the heart-shape

- Use darker powder blusher to contour the outer forehead and temples (if not covered with hair) to reduce the width of the upper half of the face. Also use it on the very point of a sharply pointed chin. Don't use it to very deeply sculpt out the cheekbone hollows.

- Highlight jaw—and chin if it is not long and sharply pointed—to add width to the lower half of the face.

- Avoid dramatically long eyelashes and rosebud lips.

- Romantic Image emphasizes the femininity of the heart-shape face, without emphasizing the heart shape. (Classic and Earthy Images emphasize the heart shape, and Glamour will too if your lashes are long and your lips small and rosebud.)

- Accessories and hairstyles are full or fuller below the ear and at the jaw and chin line than at the cheekbones or the top of the head. Avoid hair drawn up at the sides, or off the forehead (especially if you have a "widow's peak"). Bangs are helpful in camouflaging the wide forehead—especially when in conjunction with hair that is full at the jaw and chin line—except when those bangs are full, curly, and extend horizontally past the (upper half of the) head.

- Avoid v-neck and "sweetheart" necklines. Use a boat-neck neckline to reduce the pointed appearance of the chin.

Oval. The oval face shape is easiest to contour because it is considered the perfect shape and therefore requires no face shape contouring to beautify. It also requires no hair and accessory design considerations to compensate for face-shape flaws. Instead, choose makeup designs, hairstyles, and images that flatter your features while suiting your Image needs.

- Classic and Glamour Faces best emphasize the oval face.
- Hair pulled back shows off the oval face the most, while suiting both Classic and Glamour Faces. Hair pulled up at the sides gives a Romantic quality to the face.
- Wide-open necklines or close-necked, dainty collars emphasize the oval face.

For tips on contouring one or more of the features of your face, read on.

Beautifying Your Features

Here are makeup-contouring techniques to use to beautify any features that you feel could use improvement. In this chapter, you'll find many tips for contouring: wrinkles, forehead, nose, lips, chin, eyebrows, and eyes.

Cheeks are not included because there are no cheek "flaws" to require correction. If you want your cheeks to project a certain style, then look to your Image chapters, pick the style you want, and follow the technique that achieves it.

Note: If you want to make more than one improvement on a facial feature, and if that combination of techniques doesn't work together, you'll need to decide which improvement has top priority and then use the contour technique for it.

The Wrinkle

Touch up wrinkles, like those smile lines, and create a "pre-gravity" impression. Use contour-lights in the lines and shadows created by the fold or droop. This brings them forward and upward. After applying the contour-lights, blend the edges well, then powder over. When the face is finished, pick up any excess contour or powder with a cotton swab, makeup sponge, or fingertip. If a crease forms later in the day, repeat this action.

The Forehead

Forehead Not Broad Enough (and/or Too Flat or Recessed)
For the forehead to appear less narrow and more prominent, contour-light its outline. Next add a smudge of contourshadow (in this case, rouge) to the temple. Lastly contour-light with the palest possible foundation/makeup base that is suitable to your skin tone and the image you're wearing; smooth it across your forehead.

If your hair is thick, you can use full, curly bangs—extending horizontally beyond the head, if possible—instead of contouring makeup. Keep in mind that bangs are not as effective as makeup contouring.

Forehead Not High Enough
For the forehead to appear higher, place a vertical strip of contour-light down the center of the forehead, starting from the top, at the hairline, and following down the length of the nose.

Forehead Too Prominent (bulging)

For the forehead to recede, spread contour-shadow (a darker foundation/base) across the forehead. Next add a little contour-shadow (in powder form) along the hairline. Lastly contour-shadow with darker translucent powder; forehead should never shine, so touch up frequently.

Forehead Too High

To lower the forehead, spread contour-shadow (a darker foundation/base) across the forehead. Next add a little contour-shadow (in powder form) along the hairline at the top of the forehead only.

You can use a side bang or wave to soften the high forehead, allowing the contouring makeup to show.

If you were to cover the entire forehead with bangs, you would be substituting the less-effective bangs for the makeup contouring. By contrast, a short, full bang—coming only halfway down the forehead—does not totally camouflage the high forehead, and it still prevents use of the more effective contouring makeup. Instead of a full bang, try the side bang and/or contouring makeup. And remember that a high forehead is considered a beautiful sign of intelligence and refinement.

The Nose

The Sculptured Nose

Nose too short? Contour-light in a long, vertical stripe running down the center of the nose, from the bridge to the tip.

Bumps or lumps? Contour-light under or around them will help straighten them.

Too wide? Contour-light a stripe down the center of the wide area. Next contour-shadow the sides of the nose, from brow bone to nose tip, creating a more narrow, straighter-looking nose.

Too long? A touch of contour-dark (in powder form) on the end of the nose—from just below the tip—can shorten it.

Note: For nose contouring, darker foundation and powder can also be used as contour-shadows where contour products would be too obvious.

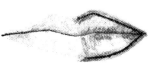

For Fuller Lips

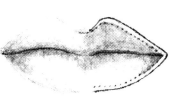

For Thinner Lips

Lips

For Fuller Lips

You can contour lips to look fuller with a non-shiny contour-light (liquid is best) applied to the center of both lips. Next, softly blend your foundation over the edges of your lips. Then define the most outside edge of your lips with a darker lipliner.

Now, carefully, with downward strokes, pat on a heavy gloss to cover all; then add your lip color, unless you're wearing Earthy Image. Only the gloss should extend over the lip-line edge. Use your darkest colors (lipliners and lipsticks) on the outsides of your lips; lightest colors on the insides.

For Thinner Lips

Use your non-shiny contour-light (liquid is best) to ring the entire outside of both your lips. Next, blend your liquid foundation over that camouflage and your lips. Keep lipliner light in color, opaque and non-shiny in finish, and as close to the inside of the lipliner edge as possible.

Don't use gloss, since shine brings features forward. If your Image requires shine, choose a moist lip balm or lipstick. Use your lightest shades of lip pencil and lipstick on the outside of your mouth.

When One Lip is Too Thin and the Other Too Full

Use white (matte liquid is best) in the center of the thin lip, and white (pencil is best) around the outside of the one that's too full. Gloss the thin one.

When Lips Are Too Long Across the Width of the Face

"Cut" lips short at the ends by covering both ends with your contour-light. Keep your lipliner pencil away from those outside corners.

The Chin

Receding Chin/Excessive Jowls

Bring jaw and chin forward by placing a line of contour-light along the jawbone.

Firm the jawline with contour-shadows under the chin, from behind the earlobe, around the underside of the jawbone, and crossing beneath the natural chinbone. Never bring it lower onto the neck than the first wrinkle or ring in the throat. Always blend with a sponge.

The Eyebrow and Eyes

Principles of the Ideal Eye and Eyebrow

When the eyes are open in a natural manner, an eye would fit in the distance between the lash line and the underside of the eyebrow. The distance between the two eyes is the length of one eye. See the following illustration, and compare it with your own eyes.

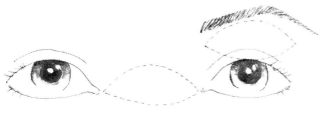

The Ideal Eye

General Eyebrow Techniques

If the eyebrow is too low, use tweezers or cuticle scissors to remove the stray brows. Apply your eyebrow makeup so that it does not weigh down the brow and bring it down toward the eye.

If your eyebrow is too high, only remove brow hairs if you must, and apply your brow makeup as heavily and low on the underside of the brow as you can to bring it down toward the eye, within the guidelines for the Image you're wearing.

Dual-Color Eyebrow Technique

At the lowest point of the brow, fill color in with your darkest accent pencil, the color of which usually matches the medium or darkest shade of your current hair color.

Next, with your eyebrow brush, brush the eyebrow up.

Use dry cake, brush-on powder eyebrow color to match the lightest or medium shade of your hair (or an accent color to complement your complexion). Brush it into the remaining uncolored eyebrow hairs, in the upper half of the brow.

Dual-Color Eyebrow Technique

Brush the pencil upward to meet and blend with the brow powder. Run your eyebrow brush the length of the brow's top edge to smooth it into the desired shape for the image you've chosen to wear. (Earthy Image does not include this step!)

Note: If your eyebrows are thick or wiry, spray your eyebrow brush with hairspray, or use setting gel on it and then brush your brows to encourage the hairs to stay in place. Prune any obvious hairs below the brow, and, if you like, even one or two of the most rebellious hairs in the brow itself, thinning it slightly, if you have truly difficult brows.

General Eye Makeup Techniques

Eye shadow is generally applied over the upper lid, on the outer half of the lower lid, in the crease above the upper lid, and then up over the outer two-thirds of the frontal (orbital) bone. Eye shadow can be used vertically or horizontally, as well as in sections of areas described. It can be powder, liquid, creme, or crayon.

An instant eye dramatizer is shadow or pencil emphasis of the crease. This gives a strong definition for the ideal eye, a well as a more finished look.

Eyeliner is generally applied along the upper and lower eyelids, as close to the eyelashes as you can manage. Eyeliner can be a line one-third, one-half, or the full eyelid length. It can be pencil, crayon, liquid, or eyebrow or eye shadow powder.

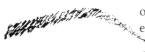

Special Eye Makeup Techniques

Under-Eye Circles. The use of only one concealer color on dark circles can give you the "raccoon-eyes" look. Instead, use your lightest cover-up, in a downward stroke, on the inner hollow of the under-eye near the tear duct at the side of the nose. Blend it on the inner half of the under-eye only, stopping in line with the pupil.

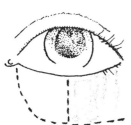

Concealed Under-Eye Circles

Next, use a slightly darker, flesh-tone concealer or base on the outer half of the under-eye area. This eliminates the look of the white-ringed eye, and the darker color doesn't make that area look puffy the way a lighter color does.

Exhausted Eyes

If you have truly exhausted eyes, splash cool water several times over your closed lids, to reduce redness and puffiness, and to temporarily tighten up the skin. Use eyedrops if desired, liquid "tears" to add moisture if they're dry; and redness-reducing drops if the cool water hasn't helped (Vitamin B6 is also wonderful to reduce redness, but it takes about a day to work—so plan ahead if you can, or use it during a stretch of irregular sleeping.)

Lastly, smooth a light layer of your palest cover-film over the entire eye socket-lids, under-eyes, outer eye/upper cheekbone area. If, after you've applied your foundation and other eye makeup, you feel that the under-eyes have the "raccoon" look or look puffy, use the technique for under-eye circles.

Eye-Brightening Blush

This lovely technique intensifies the color of your eyes, and adds a youthful, glowing look to your face. Be very subtle with this technique on Romantic and Earthy Image; it may not suit your Classic Face; it is glorious on your Glamour Face.

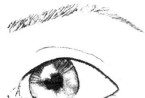

Eye-Brightening Blush

Use lipliner pencil, rouge, or lipstick on a lip brush. Place a thin line on the orbital bone, parallel from brow arch out to brow end. Then use a makeup sponge or your fingertip to lightly stipple and blend it, in place.

In horizontal eye shadowing, the brightener is usually placed on the bone just below your light, under-brow highlighter and just above the eye shadow above the crease, on the underside of the orbital bone, where it blends up to the highlighter.

Eye-Color Enhancer. You may want to draw attention to a specific color in your eye. If you have dark rims circling the iris, you can emphasize that color.

Use two colors of eye shadow: a light one the color of your inner iris, and a darker one the color of your iris rings. If you can find a colored eyeliner (often a crayon) the color of your rims, use that too for added emphasis.

If you just want to use one color of eye makeup, choosing it to match the color of your dark rims will emphasize them more than the color of your inner iris. Use neutral colors for the rest of your eye makeup.

Eye-Opener Iris Dots. This technique gets big results—big eyes! Whether you're slipping into your best candlelight face, your Glamour Image, big Romantic eyes, or perhaps wanting to open up small, narrow eyes, these iris dots are quick and easy.

Look straight ahead into the mirror; place one dot of light color (iridescent liquid is best) on the center of each eyelid. The dots are nestled practically into the lashes and allowed to dry with only the slightest patting to blur the edges.

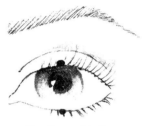
Eye-Opener Iris Dots

Doming the Eyes with Eyeliner. For big, round eyes, this technique is especially effective with Romantic and Glamour Face, or to enlarge small, narrow eyes. Begin the liner with a thin line at the inside corner of the eyelid that gradually widens over the pupil of the eye and then tapers down to a thinner line along the outer corner of the eyelid.

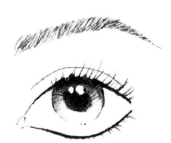
Doming the Eyes with Eyeliner

Narrowing the Eyes with Eyeliner. Narrowing the eyes is very attractive when you have a long, narrow eye, or when you want that leonine look. It's also good contouring for eyes that are too wide open, or have slack lids. Narrowed eyes tend to look piercing, sparkling, womanly; they are usually Earthy or Glamour with this technique.

Line inside the lashes and lids with pencil, or in or just above the lashes with liquid or cake liner—from the tear duct to the outer corner of the eye. (If you use liquid or cake eyeliner, you may smudge it for the "kohl" look.)

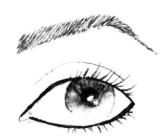
Narrowing the Eyes with Eyeliner

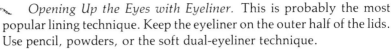

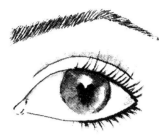

Opening the Eyes with Eyeliner

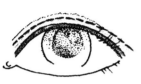

Dual-Eyeliner Technique

Opening Up the Eyes with Eyeliner. This is probably the most popular lining technique. Keep the eyeliner on the outer half of the lids. Use pencil, powders, or the soft dual-eyeliner technique.

Dual-Eyeliner Technique. You will need a liquid eyeliner as well as a pencil, crayon, or powder eyeliner for this technique. Apply the liquid liner, straight style, into the lashes on the top and bottom lids.

Use a cotton-tipped swab to blend the lower liner first, allowing the upper liner to dry slightly before smudging it with a cotton-tipped swab or your pencil or powder liner.

Next, line upper and lower lids in a normal fashion with the pencil, crayon, or powder, smoothing out the liquid and blurring it so the liquid makes the lash line look very full.

You may allow the liquid liner to show as much or as little as you like. The same is true for the second, softer-looking liner. You may even want your second liner to be a colored one, rather than a neutral.

Eyelid Basics

Are your eyelids full and prominent? Do they take away a little too much attention from your pretty eyes themselves? Just keep your upper eyelid as dark from lash to crease as you can within the Image you're wearing. If your lower lid is puffy, or prominent, use as much liner and shadow there, too, as you can in your Image. Extra mascara or even false lashes are great, especially when the Image you're wearing doesn't include much eye makeup.

Is your eyelid narrow, small, or set too far back in your head? Use the lightest colors you can, within the Image you're wearing, on the upper eyelid, from the lashes to the crease. (Don't use a shimmery product if the skin is crepey.)

When Your Eyes are not the Same Color. If your two irises are not the same color, there will usually be flecks of one similar color in both eyes. Emphasize that color, and stay in the neutral, olive, purple, or deep turquoise-grey color families. Do not use a color that appears in only one of your two eyes.

Crepey Lid Camouflage. Use creme, rather than dry, eye shadow. Use matte, rather than metallic or iridescent, eye shadows, highlighters, concealers, etc. Use non-pastel, charcoal-based colors if suited to your coloring and the Image you're wearing.

Use a gentle, stipple motion—blotting, dabbing, patting—to blend eye makeup. Dragging and pulling eye makeup around the eye traumatizes that delicate skin; as a result, the makeup doesn't apply well or look soft and natural. Not to mention the premature aging that can be precipitated by such rough handling!

Special eyebrow techniques for special brows
Brows Too Low. When the distance between the eye and the brow is less than the height of one eye, you do not have the ideal structure. This eye tends to suit the Earthy Face best.

Use a thin liner brush with your contour-lights creme or liquid, or use a white pencil to draw a thin line directly below the underside of the brow, along its entire length. Next use your most shimmery, lightest contour-light to highlight under the arch and the outer brow, down to the orbital bone. Use contour-lights on the upper eyelid, as much as you can within the guidelines of the Image you're wearing—at least a thin line near the lashes.

Conceal any shadows around the hollow near the tear-duct by the nose or any circles around the eyes. Contour the bridge of the nose with a contour-light.

Be sure the eyebrow is very well manicured, and that it is as thin and as arched as you will wear for your favorite Images.

Use pale, frosted shadows or light neutrals all over the eye and the crease. Darken the crease separately with a pencil liner. Only pale colors should be used from the lashes up to the eyebrow, except in the crease. Always make sure there is the barest hint of your whitest or lightest contour-light showing just below the brow and next to the lashes in a thin line.

This eye looks best with individual artificial lashes (not the band type), rather than just your own natural lashes.

Use the Eye-Brightener Technique under the brow.

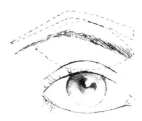 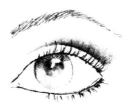

Eyebrows Too Low

Brows Too High. When the distance between the eye and the brow is more than the height of one eye, you don't have the ideal structure. This eye carries off the Glamour or Romantic Face best.

To minimize the overly spacious brow bone, three horizontal levels of color are effective. The first level is under the brow and should be light neutrals along the full length of the brow underside—either matte or shimmery whites, ivories, palest peaches, light golds.

Your second level is a dark neutral applied from the crease of the eye up to the underside of the orbital brow bone, from in line with the arch, out to the outer half of the eye.

Your third level is the color on your upper eyelid. Any variety of shadows, colors, and liners may be used to suit the Image you're wearing.

Use the Eye-Brightener Technique on that frontal bone.

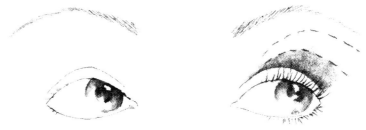

Eyebrows Too High

Special eye makeup techniques for special eyes

Eyes Too Close Together. When the distance between your two eyes is less than the length of one eye, your eyes are close-set. Vertical contour-lights on the inner half of the eye helps pull them apart. The darkest eye makeup should emphasize the outer half of the eye. Shaping the eye to appear as almond as possible adds to the illusion of wider-set eyes.

Begin all eyebrow and eye makeup slightly toward the center, rather than beginning at the inner corner of the eyelid/tear duct. To be sure of where to begin, look again at the previous ideal eye illustration. Where the eye should begin is where your eye makeup should begin even though your close-set eye does not.

Line the lashes with a smudge of color if your Image includes it; if not, use heavier mascara—or artificial lashes, if you wear them. Extend this emphasis slightly beyond the outer corner of the eyelid, out toward the temple. Don't let the upper and lower eyelid lines meet; they should run parallel out from the outer eye corner.

Eye shadow starts light at the inner third of the lids and then darkens in gradients outward until it's darkest at the outer third of the eye. It may

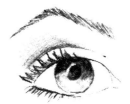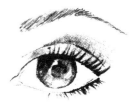

Eyes Too Close Together

be brought up toward the eyebrow at the outer third, even past the eye, if it suits the Image you're wearing.

Apply your highlighters and other lightest colors in a triangle from the tear duct to the highest point of the brow arch to finalize "pulling apart" the eyes.

Eyes Too Far Apart. When the distance between your two eyes is more than the length of one eye, your eyes are wide set. Vertical makeup design is best.

Keeping the eyelids dark, and the inner half of the crease strongly defined, brings the eyes closer together. At the outer corner of the eye, stop the eyeliner rather than drawing it longer or wrapping it around the corner. The eyeliner is widest at the inner eye, by the nose, and begins to taper over the center to its thinnest at the outer corner.

The darkest shadow is on the inner half of both upper and lower eyelids. Carry it as close to the nose, beyond the tear ducts, as will look natural and attractive. It lightens as it moves to the outer half of the eye, ending in light, shiny contour-lights from below the arch, out to the end of the brow and temple.

Begin your eyebrows closer to the nose than the tear duct if possible. Sketch in the brows with color closer to the nose than their actual beginning point. Be conservative—overcompensation will look artificial, and just a hint closer can make a lot of difference. Contour the nose to appear wider, with contour-darks.

Lashes are best emphasized from the inner corner to the center. Avoid heavy emphasis on the outer corner.

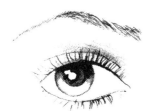 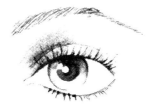

Eyes Too Far Apart

The Slim, Narrow, or Long Eye. You want to emphasize the piercing color, sparkle, and long feline feeling of this eye with eyeliner and dramatic colors. It can also look taller and rounder with vertical eye makeup contouring.

Eyeliner can be horizontal if the eye is long, and may continue out past the eyelid, toward the temple. Blur the edges to make the eye look larger.

If the eyes are merely narrow, concentrate instead on the vertical contouring: three vertical strips of shadow on the upper lid. The center third should be the lightest color, and it should shimmer. The two outer thirds can be of equal, darker intensity, or one side lighter than the other if you have close-set or wide-set eyes. Just be sure the center is the lightest of all. The Doming Eyeliner Technique is used, as well as the Iris Dot if desired. Lashes concentrate on the outer third of the narrow eye.

Eyebrows are slender and as arched as you will wear for your favorite Images; the Classic Arch, found in the Classic chapter, is the best. Brush the brows straight up from their base, and then smooth the upper edge into an arch. If eyebrows are uncompromisingly straight, they must not curve down toward the eye outer corners, but wing out toward the temples instead.

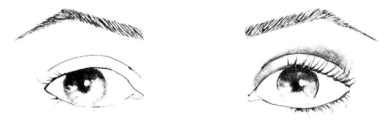

Narrow, or Long Eye

The Small Eye. Don't confuse this with the narrow eye, the deep-set eye, or the eye with the brows too close to it. The small eye is a traditionally perfectly shaped eye, but of small size. It can be made to appear larger with dark eye makeup emphasis on the outer half of the eye, and lighter contouring on the inner half.

Eyeliner is smoky and no closer to the tear duct than the pupil of the eye. Eyeliner extends slightly above and beyond the outer corner of the eye. So does eye shadow, and it wraps around the outer corner in a downward swoop.

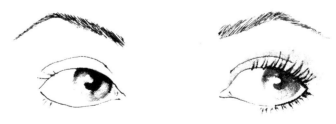

Small Eye

Never use pale, frosted colors on your eyelids; these make lids recede. Do use a thin stroke of contour-light immediately under your eyebrows, along their entire length. Use the previous Eye-Brightener Technique under the brow.

Mascara concentrates on the outer half of the eye. Eyebrows are slender and as arched as you will wear with your favorite Images. The Classic Arch, found in the Classic chapter, opens up the eye nicely. The Winged Brow, described in the Glamour chapter, is an alternative.

The Deep-Set Eye. Deep-set eyes can be very alluring when you bring the eyelid forward with lights and emphasize the crease with darker color.

Use a thin liner brush with your contour-lights creme or liquid, or use a white pencil to draw a thin line directly below the underside of the brow, along its entire length. Next use your most shimmery, palest contour-light to highlight under the arch and the outer brow, down to the orbital bone. Use sparkling, neutral contour-lights on the upper eyelid, as much as you can within the guidelines of the Image you're wearing—at least a thin line near the lashes, the full length.

Conceal any shadows around the hollow near the tear duct by the nose or any circles around the eyes. Contour the bridge of the nose with a contour-light.

Use charcoal-based colors in the crease up along the underside of the orbital bone. Bring the color up a little over the orbital bone on the outer half of the eye, making the eye appear as almond as you can. Don't use anything shimmery if the lids are crepey.

Line the lower lashes with a smudge of color or liner, extending the line slightly beyond the corner of the eye. If you aren't wearing liner, be sure to use extra-heavy mascara. Artificial lashes, whether individual or band, are usually great for bringing forward this eye.

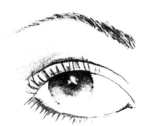 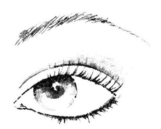

Deep-Set Eye

The Down-Slant Eye. Where the flap of eyelid skin on the outer corner of the eye makes a droop, or the shape of the eye is undesirably tipped down, use light and rouge to lift at the outer corner.

Use the heaviest and whitest contour-light in a half-circle beginning at the center of the lower eyelid and sweeping up over the corner toward the brow.

Eyeliner along the upper lid widens from the center to the outer corners of the eye. Tip it up at the outer corner. Line the lower lid to meet the outer up-tipped upper lid line. Then blur it all.

Shadow in the crease and up over the orbital bone toward the outer corner of the eye joins the up-tipped eyeliner in a square shape. See the illustration. Blend together.

Eyebrows are arched and lifted up at the corner. You may want to groom them to the Winged Brow in the Glamour chapter. Use the Eye-Brightener Technique on the spacious outer orbital bone.

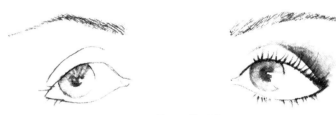

Down-Slant Eye

The Up-Tipped Eye. You may want to emphasize or minimize this feature.

To Minimize: Blend your dark eye shadow into a "wrap" around the outer corner of the eye, below the lower lashes, and tapering it gently until it reaches the inner tear duct. Then traveling from the direction of the nose, line your eyeliner to the outer corner and then tip it downward and extend it down slightly below that outer corner. Lashes are emphasized over the inner two-thirds, not the outer third.

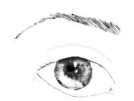 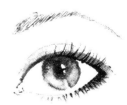

Up-Tipped Eye (Minimize)

To Maximize: Blend your eye shadow from the crease, above the tear duct, to gently widen as it fans up toward the brow's furthermost outer corner. Then apply liner on the upper and lower lids, gradually widening the upper line as you near the outside corner of the eye. Extend both upper and lower liner upward at the outer corners, trailing your brush or pencil upward to create tapered ends coming together. Lash emphasis is on the outer third of the eye.

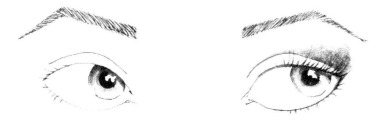

Up-Tipped Eye (Maximize)

The Short, Shallow, Smooth Eyelid. This eye has no depth or crease between lid and orbital bone. Its crease is very close to the lashes. You may create three horizontal levels with color, or you may accent the eye's shape if your skin is very pale and translucent.

To create the three-level eye, the first level of color under the brow should be a matte contour-light, which goes down only one-third of the distance between the brow and the eye. If you are emphasizing this eye shape, use a white, shimmer contour-light.

The second level should be a dark neutral, charcoal-based, or purple family color. Matte finish is better than shimmery.

The third level is the upper eyelid. It should be in a dark, charcoal- or taupe-based shadow color. Smudgy, wide eyeliner is effective and creates mystery. Line lower lashes and bring the line up to meet the upper lid color and/or liner.

Curling the lashes and using the Dual Eyeliner Technique are both beautiful on this exotic eye.

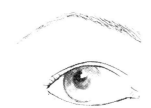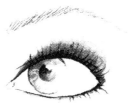

Short, Shallow Eyelid

The Oriental Eye. You may want to maximize or minimize the slant. Either way, the general guidelines are: use dark fleshtone, grey, dark gold, or medium neutrals to cover entire eyelid from lashes up over orbital bone to eyebrow. Use a medium-dark color for the second level of color, just above the entire length of the upper lid to "create" a crease. Use any choice of shadows and colors on the outer third of the lid.

To Maximize Slant: Use pale shadow on the upper and lower lids. The eye shadow on the second level, "creating" a crease, is slanted up onto the frontal bone, at the outer side of the eye, toward the temple. Use thin, dark liquid or cake eyeliner on the upper and lower lids, extended to meet upward at the outer corner. Lash emphasis is on outer third of eye.

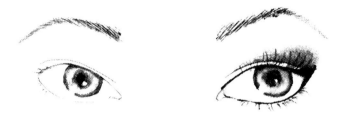

The Oriental Slant (Maximized)

To Minimize Slant: Use Dual-Eyeliner Technique and Doming shadows for the outer third of the lids, and the lash emphasis is more on the inner two-thirds. False eyelashes are especially effective.

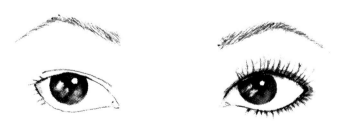

The Oriental Slant (Minimize)

The Round Eye. You may want to maximize or minimize the roundness. Romantic or Glamour Face presents the round shape well.

Extend the shadows, and the upper and lower eyeliners, to meet outside the outer corner of the eye. Heavily line the crease with a dark pencil, and extend it out slightly past the natural outer stop.

To Minimize Roundness: Remember that the thinner and darker the eyeliners, the more slanted the look, and slanting angles reduce roundness. However, this results in a more "made up" look. Don't style your eyebrows rounded.

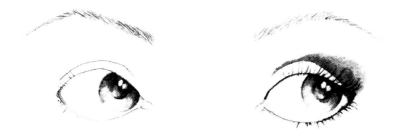

The Round Eye (Minimized)

To Maximize Roundness: It's fortunate that the Romantic Face requires a "not made up" look and rounder eye, for the rounder eye does not use the cosmetic angles. Extend the soft, smudgy liner slightly past the outer eye corners to slightly reduce the roundness if it's excessive. Curl your lashes, use the Doming Eyeliner Technique, and the Dual-Eyeliner Technique if you're not going for Romantic. Style your eyebrows rounded.

Heavy-Lidded Eye. The eyes need not be round to have heavy-lidded, "bedroom" upper eyelids. You can thin them down with dark colors.

First cover the entire eyelid with your whitest, matte contour-light. Use first liquid and then pencil liner. Thin lines cut the rounded look of the lid, and the farther out the line is extended toward the temple, the more "thinning" action it will have. Use shadow as desired.

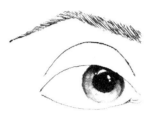 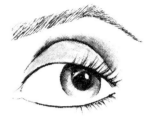

The Heavy-Lidded Eye

Bulging Eye. The bulging eye is a combination of the round eye and the heavy-lidded eye. It is usually prominent, but if it is excessively so, it may be caused by an iodine/thyroid deficiency and somewhat nutritionally correctable.

First cover the entire lid with a dark flesh base, from eyelid to eyebrow. Then use first liquid and next pencil liner. Thin lines cut the rounded look, and the farther out toward the temple they are extended, the more "thinning" action they will have.

Blend eye shadow carefully over the extended part of the upper eyelid, carrying it lightly to the line of the brow or the orbital bone. Now extend the shadows, and upper and lower eyeliners, to meet outside the outer corner of the eye. Heavily line the crease with a dark pencil or crayon, and extend it out slightly past the natural outer stop.

Lightly dust the area from the frontal bone to the eyelids with a dark, charcoal-based shadow.

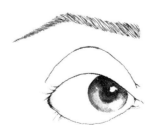 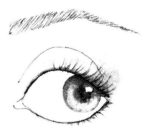

The Bulging Eye

The "Hangover" Eye. This eye is the least easy to correct until you find your most comfortable method. That has a lot to do with your age, the severity of the overhang, and whether or not the skin is crepey.

For Young, Smooth Skin: Cover the entire eye from brow to lashes with your palest, shimmery neutral over your whitest contour-light.

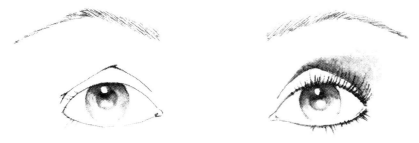

The Young, Hangover Eye

For the Mature, Crepey Overhang: Use a dark fleshtone, grey, dark gold, or medium neutral for the eyes. Avoid any shimmery cosmetics.

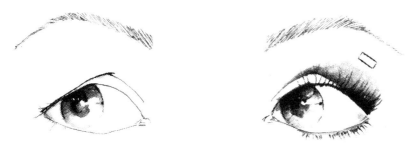

The Mature, Hangover Eye

Whether you have the smooth or the crepey eye type, line the crease heavily with a dark, creamy pencil. Choose a dark neutral or a smoky-based eye shadow for the crease, gradually fanning it up over the orbital bone, from below the arch out toward the outer corner of the eye almost up to the brow. Let it become paler in intensity the closer it gets to the brow.

Use The Dual-Eyeliner Technique on the lids. Be sure you smudge the liner so that it is very soft. Use the Eye-Brightener Technique on the orbital bone.

Eyebrows are best if meticulously groomed and arched. It gives a sharply defined look to the eye area. The Classic Arch, found in that chapter, is best. Curl your own lashes, or wear artificial ones. These eyes look best with plenty of lashes.

—Fast Face—Classic Formula

Complexion, Eyebrow, Cheekbone, Lip

Eyebrow

1 Shape, with cake eyebrow powder, into Classic Arch

2 Brush brow, and run the eyebrow brush along top of brow to return any wild hairs back to brow line

3 Highlight underneath eyebrow, its full length

Complexion

4 Perfect it: cover circles, blemishes, flaws (and lighten top eyelid centers) with light concealer stick

5 Apply light foundation with makeup sponge

Cheekbones

6 Dust face with a pad of translucent powder (loose or pressed compact)

7 Brush powder blusher into cheek hollows; blend with sponge

Lips

8 Add opaque, medium lip color—inside, or up to, lip line

Optional Touches

- A light coat of mascara
- Medium eye color in crease of the eye (just above lid)
- Lipliner pencil inside lip line (before lip color)
- Extra whisk (and later touch-ups) with face powder pad

Now turn back to Page 31 for your Check-Out!

Tear out this Classic Fast Face
guide. Hang it near your mirror.
Now, ready, get set, go!

—Fast Face—Earthy Formula

Eyebrow and Eye Emphasis, and Natural Face

Complexion

1 Do I need foundation? If so, just barely apply a warm color, with makeup sponge

2 Cover blemishes only—not freckles—with medium-tone concealer

Face Color

3 Copy the sun's kiss: cheek to cheek across the nose, using creme, gel, or liquid color

4 Lightly "sun kiss" either the temples or just above the eyebrow, or the forehead, nose and chin (your choice)

Eyebrows

5 Use brow brush to brush hairs straight up for an unruly appearance

6 Use brow powder to darken a straight line across the under-brow skin (to camouflage arch, and darken and thicken brow)

Eyes

7 Dust with smoky, earthtone shadow from lash to brow

8 Mascara the lashes: little for carefree, more heavily for exotic

Lips

9 Touch with gloss for carefree, or line lip edges with neutral pencil for exotic

Now turn back to page 63 for your Check-Out!

Tear out this Earthy Fast Face guide. Hang it near your mirror. Now, ready, get set, go!

—Fast Face—Romantic Formula

All Features Equal

Complexion

1 Quickly cover flaws and dark circles with light concealer stick
2 Blend your palest sheer foundation lightly with sponge
3 Rouge the cheek "apples"; blend well into small area with sponge
4 Dust face with translucent powder (only lightly on cheek "apples")

Eyebrows

5 Brush into rounded shape with eyebrow brush; avoid coloring them
6 Smooth your translucent powder onto rounded brows (unless already extremely light)

Eyes

7 Draw wide, domed eyeliner with sheer, neutral crayon; smudge to blur its edges
8 Add sheer, pastel color to crease; smudge to blur
9 No mascara, or barely touch light-colored mascara to top and bottom center lashes only (starry eyes)

Lips

10 Cover lightly with foundation
11 Add opaque, sheer, light color in rose or peach

Finishing Touch

12 Pat face with sea sponge wetted then squeezed "dry" (to add dewy moisture and to "set" makeup to last)

Now turn back to Page 89 for your Check-Out!

Tear out this Romantic Fast Face guide. Hang it near your mirror. Now, ready, get set, go!

—Fast Face—Glamour Formula

Complexion, Eyes, Lips

Complexion

1 Quickly perfect it: cover circles, blemishes with light-color concealer
2 Apply light-color foundation with makeup sponge

Cheekbones

3 Add slight amount of color, from hairline to no closer than outer rim of colored iris of eye

Eyes

4 Line upper and lower eyelids with crayon or pencil
5 Line crease of eye with shadow, crayon, or pencil
6 Dust on eye shadow
7 Coat lashes with mascara

Lips

8 Line lips with pencil
9 Add lip color and high gloss

Finishing Touches

10 Dust face with powder: translucent, pearlized, or translucent/pearlized mixture

   • Be sure no "L.O.T" (lipstick on teeth)!

   Now turn back to Page 114 for your Check-Out!

Tear out this Glamour Fast Face guide. Hang it near your mirror. Now, ready, get set, go!

Cosmetics List

Here are the cosmetics used to achieve the four Images in the color section.

 If you'd like to order a list of cosmetics broken down by Image and Color Key, just turn to the coupon at the back of the book.

Classic

AZIZA All Day Performing Cheekcolor—Wine
AZIZA All Day Performing Eyecolor Trio—Grey Velvet
AZIZA Silklining Pencil—Smokey Blue
AZIZA Mascara with Sealer—Black
AZIZA All Day Performing Color Sticks—Light, White
AZIZA All Day Performing Eyecolor Single—Antique Frost (jawline contour)
Estee Lauder Undercover Primer—Green
Borghese Lumina Radiant Finish Moisturizing Makeup—Italian Ivory
Max Factor Self Sharpening Automatic Eye Pencil—Light Brown
Nutri-Metics Translucent Powder—Light
Cover Girl Pressed Powder—Light
Estee Lauder Perfect Line Lip Pencil—Apple Cordial
Helena Rubinstein Lipstick—Scarlet Silk (cream)

Earthy

AZIZA All Day Performing Cheekcolor—Pink
AZIZA Natural Lustre Lip Gloss—Tawny Pink
AZIZA All Day Performing Cover Sticks—Light, White
AZIZA All Day Performing Eyecolor Single (powder shadow)—Antique Frost
AZIZA All Day Performing Eyecolor Trio—Lavender
AZIZA Silklining Pencil—Lilac
AZIZA Long & Curly Mascara—Brown
Coty All-in-One Makeup—Ivory Cane
Nutri-Metics Translucent Powder—Light

Romantic

AZIZA All Day Performing Eyecolor Trio—Copper Rose Velvet
AZIZA Silklining Pencils—Burgundy, Blue
AZIZA Really Waterproof Mascara—Black
AZIZA Natural Lustre Lip Gloss—Shiny Clear
Ultima II Pressed Powder—Medium
Elizabeth Arden Believable Color, Maximum Moisture—Ivory Beige
Elizabeth Arden Believable Color, Maximum Moisture—Cafe Beige
Estee Lauder Color Wash—Fresh Air Glow
Nutri-Metics Eyebrow Brush-n-Color—Medium Brown
Nutri-Metics Eyebrow Pencil—Blonde

Glamour

AZIZA All Day Performing Cheekcolor—Fuchsia
AZIZA All Day Performing Eyecolor Duo (powder shadow)—Crystal Frost/Delft Velvet
AZIZA Frosted Powder Pencil—Orchid Frost
AZIZA Silklining Pencils—Navy, Smokey Blue
AZIZA Long & Curly Mascara—Black
AZIZA All Day Performing Cover Sticks—Light, White
AZIZA Natural Lustre Lip Gloss—Plum Rose
Madeline Mono Lip Pencil—Hidden Sin
Germaine Monteil Creme Lipstick—Grape
Charles of the Ritz Creme Lipstick—Quiet Rose
Clinique Continuous Coverage—Creamy Glow
Revlon Touch and Glow Moisturizing Liquid Makeup—Creamy Ivory
Lancome Maquicils Mascara—Violet
Nutri-Metics Translucent Powder—Pearlucent

Index

8 Minute Makeovers Cosmetics Guide

Whether you're creating your Classic, Earthy, Romantic, or Glamour Face, your cosmetic choices are quick and easy when you use this prodect list.

The 8 Minute Makeovers Cosmetics Guide lists 33 major brand-name products. There are cosmetics for each Image and each Color Key. When you're looking for just the right makeup to create an Image for yourself, or when you're trying to find a cosmetic that best suits your own coloring, the **8 Minute Makeovers Cosmetics Guide** makes choosing your cosmetics as fast as creating your Image: 8 minutes or less!

Brands include:

Almay	Cover Girl	Germaine Monteil
Elizabeth Arden	Imperial Formula	Naturade
Artistry	Lancome	Natural Wonder
Avacare	Erno Laszlo	Nutri-Metics & Viviane Woodward
Avon	Estee Lauder	Orlane
Aziza	L'Oreal	Redken
Borghese	Alexandra de Markoff	Regalia di Notta
Charles of the Ritz	Mary Kay	Revlon
Christian Dior	Maybelline	Helena Rubinstein
Clinique	Max Factor	Shaklee Beauty Classics
Coty	Merle Norman	Ultima II

Products for each Image and each Color Key!

☐ **YES,** please send me the **8 Minute Makeovers Cosmetics Guide.** My check for $5.50 is enclosed. *(Virginia residents add 4% sales tax).* Make check payable to: 8 Minute Makeovers.

☐ Please send me a complimentary issue of *The Image Trendsletter,* the newsletter devoted to the latest trends in color, fashion, imaging, and interiors.

NAME _____

ADDRESS _____

_____ ZIP _____

Mail coupon and check to:
Cosmetics Guide
Acropolis Books Ltd.
2400 17th St., NW
Washington, DC   20009